The

# Hot Flash

## Solution

A Breakthrough Natural Program
For the Treatment of
Hot Flashes & Night Sweats.

# The
# Hot Flash
## Solution

## By Colette Bouchez

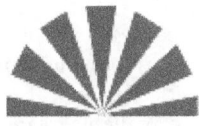

Pink Shoe Press

*London-New York*

# PSP

The Hot Flash Solution
Copyright 2009 by Colette Bouchez

Pink Shoe titles may be purchased for business or promotional use or
for special sales. For information, please write to:
PinkShoePress@aol.com
Or visit www.PinkShoePress.com

This book is not intended as a substitute for medical advice from
your physician. The reader should regularly consult with a physician
in matters relating to her health, particularly in respect to any
symptom that may require medical attention.

The author,  or  PinkShoePress  cannot be responsible for any results
obtained or derived from the information in this book. This
information is not considered medical advice and is offered only as a
guide to available treatment options.

Printed in the United States of America
10 9 8 7 6 5 4 3 2 1
First edition published 2009
Library of Congress Cataloging In Publication Data
The Hot Flash Solution/ Colette Bouchez
1.Menopause –popular works 2. Middle aged women –
Health and Hygiene.

# Dedication

To my Mom, my very best friend and
the person who taught me that you absolutely
can survive a hot flash!

To my Dad, who never had a hot flash but who
always knew what to do when Mom did.

To St. Jude – for helping me through more
than just hot flashes.

To NHL … for everything.

To all the wonderful women who have visited
YourMenopause.com and shared your stories,
your solutions, and your colorful new ways to
describe menopause: Thank you for making my
journey through this timeline so much more
interesting – & so much more fun!

And to my too fabulous Auntie Helen:
A hot flash if there ever was one!
We miss you every day.

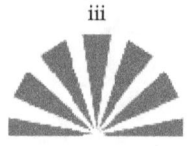

# The *Hot Flash* Solution

## By Colette Bouchez

**Contents**

**Introduction: How This Book Can Help You**

**Part One:**
**Your Changing Body & Your World**

## PART TWO:
## THE SAFE NATURAL TREATMENTS THAT CAN CHANGE YOUR LIFE

# Acknowledgments

My most sincere thanks goes to Steven Goldstein, MD, professor of obstetrics and gynecology at NYU Langone Medical Center in New York City and a member of the board of the North American Menopause Society. Dr. Goldstein's dedication to researching and treating menopause and perimenopause could never be duplicated. His "voice" is heard throughout many portions of this book.

Thanks as well to Wulf Utian, MD, president and founder of the North American Menopause Society (NAMS) an his entire staff, whose tireless work on behalf of menopause has changed the way the world looks at this time of life.

I remain indebted to the American College of Obstetricians and Gynecologists, and in particular VP Greg Philips, for never failing to help.

Special thanks to pharmacist Suzie Cohen, RPh, & nutrition guru Samantha Heller, MS, RD, who also helped launch this book on her too fabulous Sirius Radio Show. I am healthier today because of what you both have taught me!

To Julia Smith, MD, PhD, director of the Lynne Cohen Breast and Ovarian Cancer Prevention Program at the NYU – Langone Medical Center: Thank you for your friendship, for sharing your knowledge, for your unwavering dedication to women's health. The world is a better place for all women, because of you!

Finally to all the doctors and researchers around the globe who have dedicated time and energy to not only helping women survive this time passage, but end up better because of it: We appreciate everything you have done to make our lives better - just don't ask us to say thanks while we're burning up. ☺

# Signs of Menopause............

You buy an air conditioner - *for the bathroom.*

You're adding chocolate chips to your cheese omelet.

You duct tape the thermostat so no one
can raise it above 55 degrees – *in winter.*

Your husband jokes that your hot flashes are
better than solar panels. You shoot him.

The dryer has shrunk every last pair of your jeans.
The repairman tells you the dryer is working
perfectly. You call the company and insist
he be fired. Or you will shoot him.

You wonder why no one has thought of
putting estrogen in canned soup.

The Phenobarbital dose that wiped out
the Heaven's Gate Cult gives you four hours
of decent rest.

You can't believe they don't make a tampon
in size SuperDuperPlusExtra.

You can't understand why everyone you talk
to has this attitude problem lately. Crazy, isn't it? ☺

The
*Hot Flash*
Solution

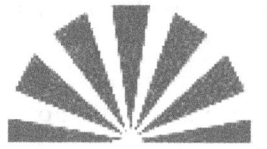

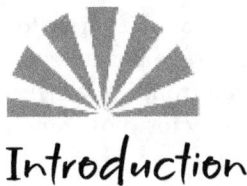

# Introduction

Dear New Friend;

In the not so distant past, I was someone very much like you, struggling through the crazy, upside down world of menopause.

Symptoms hit me out of the blue – in my early 40's – an age I thought was *much too young* to be even thinking about the change of life!

Unfortunately, I soon found out this wasn't the case. In fact, I learned that for most women the most frustrating – and sometimes devastating – symptoms of the "big change" don't actually happen at the time of menopause, when your menstrual cycle stops. They actually begin years before in a time frame known as the perimenopause. This can begin as late as your 50's or as early as your 40's – and anywhere in between.

When it does, your reproductive hormones take on a life of their own – rising, falling and turning your body chemistry upside down!

Although I had been a medical writer and reporter for many years, writing extensively about women's health - in fact many of you may know me from my articles on WebMD – still I was taken aback by just how much of an impact this was having on my life!

But as I began searching for information to help me cope, I came away feeling even more frustrated. Every book, it seems did nothing but preach the promise of hormone therapy or HRT. Indeed, even after the Women's Health Initiative Study – the first long term clinical trial of HRT – uncovered so many reasons why this should no longer be a woman's first line of defense, still I was shocked to discover that so much of the information being offered to women in books, in magazines, and on the Internet, continued to point to HRT as the ultimate solution.

Nowhere was this more true than when it came to treating what had become my most troubling symptoms: Hot flashes and night sweats. And it was a problem I soon learned affects up to 75% of all women.

Of course, for some women birth control pills, or HRT used for a very short time at a very lose dose can be an enormous *temporary* bridge.

But from my perspective the problem has always been what happens when you stop? For most women, the flashes come flashing back – and they *still have* to find a way to cope. Moreover, many women undergoing treatment for breast cancer must also deal with hot flashes – no matter their age.

In fact, while hot flashes can start in the years leading up to menopause – as early as age 40 - they can also continue for many years after, so that sometimes even women in their 60's and 70's can still get the "the burn".

Yikes! Was I to endure 20 or even (gulp!) 30 years of feeling like my hair is on fire and my pajamas are going to explode?

Not this girl.

OUT OF FRUSTRATION – CAME ANSWERS

Convinced I was going to find the answers, I set out on a two-year research journey, one that took me to every expert on the subject of menopause I could find. I talked to doctors, scientists, naturopathic physicians, acupuncturists, nutritionists, exercise physiologists – if there was anyone with a menopause thought in their in head, I wanted to hear it!

I coupled this with hours and hours reading over research papers, looking not only in traditional medical journals, but alternative ones as well. The end result: I learned more about perimenopause and menopause – and all the symptoms and changes that a woman's body goes through – than I ever dreamed possible.

Ultimately, I learned so much that in 2005 I published my findings in a book titled:

*Your Perfectly Pampered Menopause:Health, Beauty and Lifestyle AdviceFor The Best Years of Your Life."*

And I knew instantly I had struck a chord in the hearts of women everywhere! Not only did critics hail my book as the "New Bible of Menopause" but thousands of women from all over the world wrote to share the stories of their own menopause journey, and to tell me how much my book helped them along the way.

It was truly one of the most gratifying journalism projects I've ever undertaken! And if you get a chance I think you'll really enjoy reading it.

THERE WAS STILL MORE TO LEARN. . .

As complete a book as *Your Perfectly Pampered Menopause* is, and as much new and important information as it contains, there was still one area where I just wasn't satisfied. And oddly enough, it had to do with the reason I started that first journey to begin with: Trying to find a treatment for hot flashes that really worked!

At the time, I wrote as much as I could possibly find on the topic, and offered as many solutions as I could uncover. And while some of the remedies featured in the book helped me, and I was definitely feeling better in general, the truth was, I was still having hot flashes – and I still wasn't sleeping as well as I knew I should or could.

Well of course my doctor was right there with the old prescription pad, saying "I told you so", just waiting for me to give in. But I didn't. Instead, I set out on a second research journey – this one dedicated to just one purpose: *Find The Hot Flash Solution!*

I would be the Indiana Jones of Menopause - and I wouldn't stop until I had an answer!

## Help Without Hormones … Possible?

Among the very first things I discovered was how much research had taken place and how many more options were now available, in just the two years since I had published my last book.

There were new studies on how vitamins, herbs, nutrients, and diet could make a difference in hot flashes, plus new research on stress, exercise, and relaxation, even the role of aromatherapy. And all of it was good, important data that I became very eager to share.

But through the course of doing all this research, I stumbled upon something else – something so new, something so entirely different, and something I knew no one else had thought about before.

What I discovered: The important role that a woman's lifestyle plays in not only how well she copes with hot flashes, but also in orchestrating the severity and the frequency of many menopause symptoms. . Moreover, I discovered just how personal these effects could be.

For example, in some women alcohol can have a major influence on the severity of hot flashes – but the level of that influence can be dramatically different in every woman.

I discovered how certain foods could make night sweats worse for some – and yet have no impact on others. I even found research concerning the way in which our choice of clothing, specifically the fabrics we choose, can play a role in bringing on a hot flash and making it last longer – and I'm not just talking about dressing in layers!

In fact, while I knew that the mechanisms involved in causing hot flashes were indeed physiologic in nature, I was astounded to discover how much of an impact these personal lifestyle factors could really have.

Now … if I could only find a way to tie it all in together so that women everywhere could find relief!

Well I'm happy to say I did find a way! (I'll bet you knew I would!) And that answer is my patent-pending Hot Flash Solutions Lifestyle Diary - a fun, easy system that allows every woman to zero in on the personal lifestyle factors impacting not only her hot flashes and night sweats but her entire quality of life during this unique and special time.

Using my system you'll begin to immediately understand how your personal world influences your perimenopause and menopause symptoms – and you'll begin to discover which simple changes will make the most difference in how you feel. Within approximately 7 to 14 days you will have determined your Personal Hot Flash profile – or PHF - and be well on your way to eliminating the lifestyle triggers that can impact you the most!

You'll find a full explanation of how to use the diary in Chapter 5 – plus you'll find a sample diary page.

You can also visit TheHotFlashSolution.com & download a color chart that prints out on standard size copy paper.

Certainly, for many of you, the life style changes you'll learn about in Part One will be all you need to reduce your hot flashes & night sweats to a level you can easily tolerate.

But for those who still need more help there is Part Two - the single most comprehensive guide to the safest, most natural ways to alleviate hot flashes and night sweats *without prescription drugs*. You'll discover what medical studies show really works, - *and what doesn't!* You'll even find important health precautions to keep you extra safe!

Ultimately, you'll have everything you need to take control of your menopause symptoms once and for all! In fact, while this book is focused on hot flashes and night sweats, don't be surprised if the same steps you take to eliminate these problems also help reduce or eliminate many other related symptoms as well!

So, sit back, relax, and put your feet up! What you're about to learn can change your life. Or, at least make it seem like it's a lot less hot in here! ☺

Warm Regards;

*Colette Bouchez*

PS: I'd love to hear how The Hot Flash Solution has helped you. Or, you have one or two of your own I haven't yet discovered, please let me know! Write me at : RedDressDiary@aol.com

# Part One:

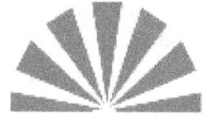

# Your Changing Body

# & Your World

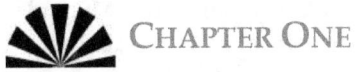 CHAPTER ONE

# Understanding Your Changing Body

As the saying goes, there are only two sure things in life: Death and taxes. Well I'd like to add a third: If you're woman, it's hot flashes!

Indeed, as the infamous and inevitable part of the life stage we call menopause, the "hot flash" has come to signify a kind of feminine *rite of passage* – one that binds of us together in a way that even the bra burning - feminine freedom movement of the sixties could not do.

But in reality, it's not actually menopause that kicks off this and a variety of other symptoms we associate with this time of life. Indeed, the true medical definition of menopause means no menstrual period for at least 12 months – no bleeding, no spotting, no little "oops" for a day or two. And truthfully, by the time you get to *that stage*, a good deal of the symptoms associated with this time of life are actually pretty manageable – and many disappear completely. And life after menopause …it can be pretty good.

Without the worry and fear of an unexpected pregnancy – not to mention the craziness of PMS and the bloating and pain of menstrual cramps – arriving at the gates of menopause can be a very freeing experience, often becoming the springboard to a brand new life. For those of you who regularly visit my blog RedDressDiary.com, you already know some of the terrific benefits that being *grown up – and not old* - can offer!

But the time leading up to the "Big M' … *maybe not so great.* In fact, while legendary symptoms such as hot flashes and night sweats are always linked to the term "menopause", in reality, they start much earlier, during a time known as the "perimenopause." This can begin as early as age 40 or as late as your early 50's and from a symptom point of view it can definitely be among the most trying times in a woman's life.

## UNDERSTANDING PERIMENOPAUSE

If you're like most women you probably began to notice the first signs of perimenopause somewhere around your 40th birthday. Among the most common are changes in your monthly cycle. You know it as "irregular periods": Some months your flow is exceptionally light, other times uncharacteristically heavy. There may be fewer - or more - days between each cycle, often interspersed with several months of "regular", periods that arrive on time.

But changes in your monthly cycle are not the only thing that's different. Because this is also the time when many women begin to experience a variety of related symptoms – including not only hot flashes and night sweats, but also  memory problems, fatigue, anxiety, mood swings, and a  sex drive  that can vacillate from "Gotta have it now" to " Don't you dare touch me" – sometimes within a single day! You may also feel weepy and emotional one moment, and mad as heck the next – *and almost always ready to take on a good fight!*

So…what's happening - and why?   The short answer is your ovaries are getting old!   As a result, your reproductive hormones are no longer working the way they should.

But before you can fully appreciate *what this means* – and how and why it's causing your symptoms - it's important to understand a little bit about how your ovaries function throughout  your reproductive life .

## HOW YOUR OVARIES WORK

From puberty onward, much of your reproductive activity revolves around the production of estrogen and progesterone – two of your key reproductive hormones.  They're made primarily in your ovaries.

The other two hormones of note are FSH (follicle stimulating hormone) and LH (luteinizing hormone), both of which are manufactured in your brain.

Rounding out your reproductive biology are your egg follicles or "seeds".  These are tiny sacs within each ovary that are filled with the biological material necessary to grow into an egg.  How and why that happens is the direct result of your monthly menstrual cycle – which starts the moment puberty arrives. The activity goes something like this:

- At the start of each cycle, estrogen levels are low. This sends a message to your brain to manufacture FSH – the hormone which stimulates egg follicles to grow.

- As the growth phase occurs, one follicle pulls ahead and begins to develop into an egg. This activity causes your estrogen level to rise quite dramatically. When it reaches a specific point, your brain releases LH – the hormone which prompts that developed egg to pop from your ovary – a process known as ovulation.

- As soon as this happens, the shell which housed the egg begins producing progesterone, which, together with estrogen creates a spongy nest of blood vessels inside your uterus. If your egg is fertilized by your partners sperm that "nest" becomes the womb where your fertilized egg attaches and begins to grow. To nourish it, both estrogen and progesterone levels remain high.

- If, however, no fertilization takes place, levels of both hormones drop rapidly. It is this rapid drop in hormone levels that cause the spongy lining inside your uterus to break down and be shed. This shedding process becomes the basis of your menstrual bleed.

If you are in basic good health, this "monthly cycle" repeats itself over and over throughout all your reproductive years.

As you begin to age, however, your ovaries age as well – and as a result some of these steps begin to change.

## HOW YOUR OVARIES AGE

While you may look 35 on the outside, I can assure that once you hit 40, and certainly by age 45, your ovaries are showing your *true age!* The first thing that happens: Some of your egg follicles have died off, while what's left behind becomes much less responsive to FSH. In short, they simply don't get the "signal" to grow as easily or as often as they did in the past. The end result is that ovulation no longer occurs on a regular, monthly basis.

In fact, sensing that no follicle growth is occurring frequently your brain responds by pouring out still more FSH – in an effort to get things moving again. While sometimes it works – at some point it stops working - which is one reason that high levels of FSH can be a sign that your body has begun the process leading up to menopause.

In any event, by the time you are in your 40's, you are probably ovulating only about 6 to 8 times a year- instead of the normal 12 times. Without regular ovulation, there is no regular, consistent estrogen production. As a result the level of this hormone begins to waiver – sometimes estrogen is high, sometimes it's low.

But this isn't the only hormonal change that's occurring. Without ovulation your body can't produce adequate amounts of progesterone. So that means whatever estrogen you are producing becomes "dominant". This creates an imbalance similar to what occurs during PMS – one reason so many of the symptoms of perimenopause are so similar.

In fact, while most women believe that all their perimenopause symptoms are the result of low estrogen, the truth is that many problems – including mood swings, sore breasts and changes in sex drive – primarily occur because estrogen and progesterone are no longer in balance. Thus you can end up feeling much the way younger women do when they have PMS. The only difference here: While PMS usually lasts no more than 5 to 10 days, perimenopause symptoms can continue for much longer, and occur randomly and more frequently.

## HOT FLASHES & HORMONE IMBALANCE

Although many women say their first and most easily recognizable sign of perimenopause *is* the irregular cycles, it's not just your V zone that is impacted by hormonal changes. Indeed, there are hormone receptors throughout your body – cells that need progesterone, but more importantly estrogen, to function properly.

While most of your estrogen receptors reside in your breast, uterus and ovaries, there are also some located in your gut, urinary tract, skin, bones, liver, brain, blood vessels, even your central nervous system. So, it's easy to see how you can feel the effects of a hormonal imbalance body-wide. It's also why you can feel so good when your hormones are in balance! Indeed, when your ovaries are functioning at peak capacity and eggs are being regularly made, there is more than enough estrogen available to meet the needs of all cells that require it. So, for the most part, your body is humming along – and you feel good.

But as your ovaries age – and ovulation declines - there is simply less estrogen to go around. And that can leave your receptor cells playing a kind of "hormonal musical chairs"! Sometimes a receptor cell will be filled, other times, it won't. And it is precisely this kind of waxing and waning activity that doctors now believe triggers the entire cascade of perimenopause symptoms – including hot flashes and night sweats.

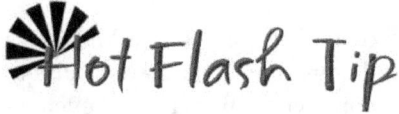

For quick hot flash relief when you're on the go carry a migraine cool patch! These ultra thin portable gel packs provide instant cool with no refrigeration needed. Just unwrap it and place it on the back of your neck , or on the inside of your elbow or wrist to instantly cool you down and reset your thermostat.

Brands include Wellpatch and Kool Patch .

 CHAPTER TWO

# Understanding A Hot Flash: What You Need To Know

According to research, up to 75% of all middle aged women experience hot flashes. And while it's not common, up to 10% are still experiencing "the burn" *up to 15 years after their period stops!*

But what exactly is a hot flash?

For most women it begins with a kind of "aura "that occurs just before the burn starts . Frequently this includes a somewhat dramatic or even frightening increase in heart rate. According to NYU professor Steve Goldstein, MD, it's not uncommon for a woman's pulse to hit 150 beats per minute during a hot flash. If you are prone to panic attacks, you might also feel a sudden increase in anxiety, which is triggered when your heart rate increases.

Following this, most women feel a sudden surge of heat. It usually begins in the face and spreads quickly to the neck and chest. Sometimes the skin will actually appear red.

You may also get a feeling of tightness or constriction in your chest muscles. Be aware, however, that these can also be signs of an impending heart attack, so if your symptoms don't fade within 5 to 10 minutes or if they are accompanied by nausea and dizziness that also doesn't go away quickly, do seek immediate medical attention.

## WHAT CAUSES A HOT FLASH?

Although hot flashes have been going on since, well, there have been women on earth to have them, surprisingly, the first study on this uniquely feminine phenomenon wasn't even published until 1975 – appearing in a little known publication called the *Journal of Applied Physiology*.

It was here that research finally documented what actually happens when a flash occurs. Among the first things noted was a change in skin temperature – an increase when the flash starts, followed by a rapid decrease as the flash subsides. The cardiovascular system also gets looped into the reaction, causing your heartbeat to increase by about 13% as each flash begins. As you just read, that can mean an increase up to 150 beats per minute for a short period of time.

Eventually doctors came to classify this cascade of activity as "vasomotor instability". This means your blood vessels are contracting and expanding in an unpredictable fashion, without any justifiable cause.

But why is this happening? Initially doctors believed a reduction in estrogen was the primary cause of hot flashes – an idea that actually gave birth to the concept of estrogen replacement therapy, the first form of menopausal hormone therapy. While it seemed to work – at least in theory - there was one piece that didn't fit into the puzzle – namely, until puberty *all girls* have low estrogen levels and none of them have hot flashes.

Moreover, during the third trimester of pregnancy – a time when estrogen levels are generally high - many women experience hot flashes – more evidence that estrogen alone could not be the whole cause.

Still, because hot flashes occur during a time when a woman's estrogen levels *are changing*, the connection was hard to deny. Ultimately researchers came to understand that it was not so much the level of estrogen that mattered most, but rather the erratic, *continually changing* level that was at the heart of most perimenopause symptoms – particularly hot flashes and night sweats. What happens – and why?

Dancing Hormones And Hot Flashes

Today many experts believe it all centers on the hypothalamus - a tiny gland located deep within the brain that controls body temperature. Not coincidentally, the hypothalamus is filled *with estrogen receptors.*

Normally, this gland works in a very predictable way to control your body temperature. For example, when you become overheated – from exercise, or when you're simply racing around in warm temperatures - this gland picks up on the activity, and sends a message to your body that your core temperature is rising.

Your body responds to that message by causing your blood vessels to widen or "dilate" which in turn allows some of that core heat to *gradually* be released. That's usually when you start to perspire - another natural way your body adjusts your core temperature and helps you to cool down.

Once your core temperature returns to normal, your blood vessels constrict to conserve body heat. This keeps your body temperature from dropping too low, and allows you to stop perspiring. Usually, before long, you feel cooler and more comfortable.

But during the perimenopause, the estrogen-sensitive hypothalamus begins acting in a very erratic and unusual way. Indeed, without the benefit of regular and consistent estrogen stimulation, your entire temperature regulating system appears to go somewhat out of control.

HOW YOUR BODY TEMPERATURE GOES AWRY

It begins when your hypothalamus gets the wrong message – believing that you are overheated even when you're not. When this occurs it sends out a powerful biochemical SOS to tell your body to do whatever is necessary to cool you down. Your body's natural response to that message is an extremely rapid dilation of blood vessels – an activity that causes you to rapidly release a large amount of heat quickly.

Ironically, it is this "cool down" signal that is actually responsible for your hot flash!

Indeed, instead of the gradual release of heat that normally occurs when you are overheated from activity, the heat release that occurs during a hot flash is so rapid and intense you actually experience the entire event through your skin. It's what you already know as that spreading sensation of warmth that often starts in your face and neck and quickly goes to your chest, arms, and trunk. Your skin may feel hot to the touch – and even turn red.

As you probably also know, usually within 5 to 10 minutes your brain figures out that the message it sent your body was wrong. Moreover, since your core temperature was never really elevated to begin with, your body is now in danger of becoming too cold!

To compensate your brain sends out another urgent SOS telling your blood vessels to immediately stop releasing heat. This in turn causes them to rapidly constrict, allowing your flash to stop. Because, however, you have discharged *so much* body heat so quickly, the "burn" is often followed by "the chill", sometimes to the point of getting the shivers. While not all women experience this aspect of a hot flash, many do report feeling cold after the heat subsides.

Moreover, while some women experience one hot flash at a time, with hours or even days in between, others can experience "multiple flashes", sometimes interspersed with the chills, one occurring right after another.

Some may feel just continuous flashes with no chills – so it feels like one long hour of burning - while others can get flashes of short duration, but they occur frequently – sometimes as often as 10 times per day. The point is every woman can experience a flash in a slightly different way, with reactions varying from day to day.

## WHAT CAUSES NIGHT SWEATS

For many years doctors believed that a "night sweat" was a symptom unto itself – something apart and different from a hot flash that occurs during the day.

But today, the consensus of medical opinion is that a night sweat is simply the compilation of a lot of hot flashes that occur while you sleep.

Although initially the flashes don't wake you, they do interfere with your ability to experience deep sleep - one reason many women going through perimenopause often feel so fatigued, even if they appear to get enough hours of sleep.

Eventually, however, this hot flash activity does wake you, usually at the point where you are drenched in sweat.

Certainly, the circuitry of the hypothalamus - and the influence of hormone receptors – appears to be the major physiologic reason behind both hot flashes and night sweats.

But as you will begin to discover in the chapters that follow, there are also many lifestyle factors that can play an important role - frequently exacerbating this physiologic activity or sometimes even acting as the initial trigger that sets a flash in motion.

And while these precipitating lifestyle factors can be slightly different for every woman, the good news is that once you identify yours, taking control of hot flashes and night sweats is easier than you think!

Even better news: For many women getting these two symptoms under control can also help alleviate some other perimenopause symptoms especially those linked to a lack of deep sleep. And in the following chapters you'll learn how to do that as well!

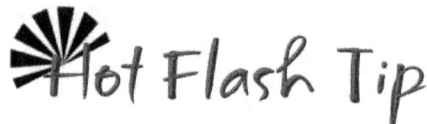 Hot Flash Tip

To reduce your night sweats

try wearing socks to bed!

Here's why: When your feet are warm

it sends a message to your brain that your

body temperature is just right –

and that in turn can help stabilize your

"thermostat" so you don't have those

wild swings in heat release.

 CHAPTER THREE

# Hot Flashes & Your Personal World

It's you've ever had a menopause discussion with your best friend – or even your doctor - then you already know that no two women experience the change of life in the exact same way. While for some the main issues *are* hot flashes and night sweats, for others it can be memory loss, mood swings, sleep loss or even a variety of seemingly unrelated aches and pains.

For some the symptoms are mild and barely worth talking about; for others they can be debilitating. This broad spectrum of experiences has led many women to wonder why, if we're all going through the same physiologic changes, we all don't experience that change in the same way.

Well one reason has to do with heredity. Programmed into your DNA - right there next to how many bad hair days you're going to have - Mother Nature has created some genetic links to menopause. In fact, when your symptoms start, when they end, and what goes on in between can be greatly influenced by your genetics - one reason why many daughters experience menopause in a way that is similar to what their mother experienced. And many sisters also have similar experiences.

But as research has now shown, it's not just heredity that determines how your perimenopause symptoms unfold. Today doctors now know that your personal health, your lifestyle, and your environment can also play a huge role. (And no, I'm not talking global warming! ☺ )

In fact, the way each of us lives our life can not only shape our risk profile for a variety of diseases, it also appears to impact how easy- or how difficult – our midlife transition turns out to be. And nowhere is this truer than when it comes to hot flashes and night sweats.

While research in this area is, admittedly, still pretty new, there is a growing body of evidence to show that what we do from day to day, including what we eat and drink, our stress levels, how much or how little we exercise, the medications we take - even certain factors in our immediate environment - can, on their own, or in unison, make our menopause time much harder – *and hotter* – than it needs to be!

But at the same time, remember, when it comes to the "changes", there are few hard and fast rules. So that also means there is no *one food,* no *one medicine*, no *one environmental factor* that we can point to as a definitive link to hot flashes and night sweats – or any other menopause or perimenopause symptom.

That said, there are lots of places to look for the *usual suspects* - and lots of individual lifestyle factors that can make a difference as well. The key lies in figuring out which of those factors impacts you the most – and then learning how to avoid or eliminate them – or at the very least reduce their impact.

To help you do just that I've created my brand new, patent-pending Hot Flash Solutions Diary. In short, it's a way of keeping track of your hot flashes *and your hot flash triggers* that allows you to quickly and easily identify which personal lifestyle and environmental factors may be behind *your worst symptoms*.

Then, by changing, rearranging or modifying those factors, you can not only reduce the number of hot flashes and night sweats you experience, but in some cases figure out how to nearly eliminate them.

And a little later in this book you'll find the **Hot Flash Solutions Lifestyle Diary Chart** – along with easy to follow instructions. You can also download and print out a larger copy of the chart which is available free of charge at: TheHotFlashSolution.com.

But before you begin looking for your personal hot flash triggers, it's important that you learn a little about some of the more common lifestyle and environmental factors that could be affecting you.

These are factors that many women find they have in common, so they might be true for you as well. In addition, they can also help get you thinking in the right direction, so you are clearer on where to look for your own personal hot flash triggers.

## FOODS AND HOT FLASHES

Among the more important influences on your hot flash physiology is your daily diet. While research in this area is just beginning to blossom, there is certainly good evidence to show that for many women, daily food choices can make a significant difference in how well they cope with hot flashes and night sweats – as well as influencing how they feel overall.

Perhaps more importantly, outpacing the research right now is the number of anecdotal reports made by women themselves, concerning how the foods they eat seem to influences how they feel during this time of life.

Later in this book you'll read about some of the foods that science shows – and many women believe - can help *reduce* the risk of hot flashes.

But for right now I'd like you concentrate on those foods that have at least the potential to bring on the burn.

Of course, as in any health condition, the dietary impact on menopause symptoms can be very personal. And, if you use my Hot Flash Solutions Diary to chart your personal hot flash triggers, you may soon have your own "hot list" of the foods that affect you the most. But to help get you thinking in the right direction now, what follows are some of the foods that, in many women, will trigger hot flashes & night sweats. If they prove to be behind your symptoms as well, the quickest relief will come if you eliminate them from your diet.

But what if they are  true favorites you just can't live without? Try reducing the amount you consume, or if there is more than one food linked to your symptoms, try not to eat them all during the same meal. This will reduce the overall impact,   plus in lesser amounts they may cause fewer or no problems.

## HOT FLASH FOODS TO AVOID

**CAFFEINE** – Whether in coffee, tea, cola, or chocolate, caffeine is a stimulant that can raise blood pressure and increase heart rate. And it's these physiologic changes, say experts ,that  in some women can trigger a hot flash. While you probably don't have to cut caffeine out completely, you should pay attention to your personal threshold – the amount you can safely consume without inciting a flash. Again, charting your personal reactions will help you find your limit.

**HOT BEVERAGES** – Any hot liquid – be it cup of herbal tea, a bowl of chicken soup, or a mug of hot cocoa – can temporarily impact body temperature. In doing so it can confuse the already confusing messages your brain is sending to your body about your core temperature. If your hot drink also happens to contain caffeine, it could have an even greater impact on your hot flashes.

**ICY COLD BEVERAGES** – When you're hot and sweaty nothing sounds better than a cold drink. And for most folks it can offer relief.  But for the menopause woman any abrupt change in body temperature can be enough to trigger a flash – and a very cold drink can do that. To reduce the impact, try leaving the ice out of your soda or water, and then let it sit for a few minutes before drinking it. This will help moderate the temperature. If you're out socially and your only beverage choice is an ice-packed drink, sip it slowly, holding it in your mouth for a few seconds before swallowing. This will also help moderate the temperature change.

**Hot Spicy Foods** - Much like caffeine, very hot spicy foods can trigger a spike in blood pressure and heart rate that can ignite a cascade of physiologic changes linked to hot flashes. For some women even mild spices like white pepper can jar temperature-regulating mechanisms and trigger a hot flash. For others, flashes don't get hot and steamy until they bite into a jalapeno pepper. So, often your reaction is tempered by what your body is used to. Either way, pay attention to any spice-flash connection to find the threshold that's best for you.

**Alcohol** – A little is good – even during menopause. A lot is bad - bad for your general health and maybe bad for your hot flashes. Research has shown that alcohol can cause an immediate spike in blood levels of estrogen, followed by a rapid drop. It's that up-and-down motion that can trigger the flash – or even a mood swing you aren't expecting, or didn't experience from alcohol before this time of life.

**Sweets** - Eating sweet foods can give an immediate temporary boost to your metabolism – and that creates heat. Sometimes it's enough of a fire to trigger a hot flash – or certainly make one you've already got feel worse or last longer. While you don't have to give up sugar completely, you may find that reducing your intake is helpful. More important, be mindful of where your personal cut off point is. For most women one or two teaspoons won't make much difference. Get into the 12 spoonfuls found in a can of soda and you could end up red–in-the-face a lot more often! **Also note:** White flour is metabolized much like sugar, and rapidly turns into glucose soon after it's ingested. So also consider the flash impact of foods that have little sugar but a lot of white flour such as white bread, rolls, and   pasta.

ARTIFICIAL SWEETENERS - The evidence is clearly anecdotal and no medical studies have found any links between artificial sweeteners like aspartame (NutraSweet) and hot flashes. That said, there are now so many isolated reports on the Internet directly from women who claim their hot flashes are made worse by this and other similar "fake sugars" that it's worth mentioning. If you consume a lot of products using artificial sweeteners and you get a lot of hot flashes, it might be worth a personal investigation to see if they could be contributing to your symptoms.

FOOD ADDITIVES/MSG (monosodium glutamate) - An amino acid that is often used as a flavor enhancer particularly in Asian cuisine, MSG has been known to impact vaso-motor activity, including causing rapid dilation of blood vessels. Since this activity is similar to what occurs during a hot flash, there are a number of experts who believe MSG can act as a trigger, particularly in women who may be sensitive to the effects. By law, all foods containing MSG sold in the United States must state that on the label.

However, many food purists argue this ingredient is often "hidden" by listing it under alternate names such as hydrolyzed vegetable protein (HVP), autolyzed or hydrolyzed plant protein (HPP or APP), autolyzed yeast, Sodium caseinate, Calcium caseinate, and numerous other terms. Moreover, restaurants aren't required to reveal if they use MSG or any of its derivatives, so you may have to speak up and ask if it's on the menu. If MSG has caused other symptoms for you in the past – like dizziness or a headache – then it's more likely to trigger or exacerbate a hot flash as well.

SULFITE – A food preservative that can cause hot flashes in some women, sulfite is commonly found in canned tuna, crackers, dehydrated foods, some frozen foods and many "crunchy' snacks. It can also be listed under alternative names such as sodium sulfite, sodium bisulfite, sulfur dioxide, or any ingredient that ends in *sulfite*. Check ingredient labels to know for sure.

## SMOKING AND HOT FLASHES

I'm certain you are well aware of how dangerous smoking is, particularly for women. Not only does it increase your risk of heart attack and stroke, but because women's blood vessels are much smaller than men's, problems occur at a much younger age.

Smoking also increases the risk of several female cancers including breast cancer – and if that were not enough it can also decrease bone density, setting you up for a weakened skeleton and possibly even severe disability as you age.

And for many of us, the absolute most devastating effect of cigarettes is that they age the skin! Women who smoke get far more wrinkles than those who don't – and they start earlier!

But for many women the most surprising fact about smoking is that it can increase hot flashes! They can begin at a younger age, last for more years, and feel much worse – and there is some evidence to show that smoking may be a direct trigger, causing a hot flash to occur.

In one study published in the journal *Menopause*, researchers from the University of Michigan found that women who smoked reported twice as many severe hot flashes as women who didn't. Smokers who were overweight reported 7 times more hot flashes than thin smokers!

Still, regardless of what you weigh, if you smoke, try to stop. You'll look and feel better almost immediately, and your hot flashes may decrease dramatically as well.

## ALLERGIES AND HOT FLASHES

From food to fragrance from flowers to fabrics to formaldehyde, almost anything is capable of inciting an allergic response. For many, part of the sensitivity reaction involves hot flashes. While an allergy – related hot flash occurs for an entirely different reason, still, they play a role in your overall menopause hot flash experience.

And while it's rare that an adult develops a *sudden* allergy to any particular food or substance, what can move front and center during mid-life are *sensitivity reactions* you might not have experienced, or noticed before.

Causing a mild to moderate reaction – including hot flashes - sensitivities can grow worse during the perimenopause, and when you are exposed to multiple sensitivities. For example, studies show a food sensitivity that lays dormant much of the year can suddenly be activated when exposure to another sensitivity occur, such as a related tree pollen.

Moreover, while you may have had a mild sensitivity reaction to something in the past – including mild facial flushing - it may have gone almost unnoticed until this time in your life. That's when hormone-related hot flashes may be combining with allergic sensitivity related hot flashes to make both problems feel worse.

The good news is that by tracking down the cause of your allergic hot flashes – and eliminating them - you may be able to reduce the severity of your hormonal hot flashes.

But even if you can't – or don't want to - eliminate a hot flash sensitivity trigger, like a favorite food for example, simply identifying it can help you avoid it at key times, when you're trying to minimize the occurrence of hot flashes.

And while almost anything is capable of kicking off an allergy-related hot flash sensitivity (and again, the chart later in this book will help you track your personal triggers) you should pay special attention to foods, flowers, plants, as well as environmental fragrances, including your own perfume.

Other sources to consider include: Room fresheners; laundry detergent; chemical odors from home furnishings such as a new carpet, carpet padding or upholstery; furniture made from pressed wood or MDF; office chemicals such as printer ink, chemicals from a fax machine or fax paper; office furnishings; dry cleaning chemicals and residues left on clothes; home decorator or craft supplies (paint, glue, etc); and magazines or newspapers printed with colored inks. Any and all can initiate an allergic hot flash.

## MEDICINES AND HOT FLASHES

Unlike hot flashes caused by an allergy or sensitivity, hot flashes that result from medications are usually due to side effects. Hot flashes can also develop when medications "clash" – two drugs come together to influence your vaso motor activity in a way that results in a hot flash.

While these aren't the same as hormone-related hot flashes, the experience is similar – and because it involves vaso-motor activity it can actually bring on, or certainly exacerbate a menopause flash.

So, if you are taking any prescription or over-the-counter medications on a regular basis, or if you start any new drugs during your perimenopause or menopause, do remember to ask your doctor if hot flashes could be a side effect. If this turns out to be the case, there may be a different medicine that you can take instead.

**CAUTION:** *Never stop any medications without talking to your doctor first – even if you think they arecausing hot flashes – doing so could prove dangerous.*

According to pharmacist and author Suzy Cohen, R.Ph, the drugs that may cause a hot flash include:

•Calcium channel blockers – medications used to treat high blood pressure.

•Antidepressant medications known as SSRIs drugs like Prozac, Effexor, Cymbalta and Sarafem.

•Estrogen Receptor Drugs such as Tamoxifen, often prescribed breast cancer, Evista or Boniva used to treat osteoporosis.

•Niacin, the B vitamin, which in high doses can cause the skin to flush.

•Aromatase inhibitors – Cancer treatment drugs including Aromasin, Arimidex and Femara.

•Migraine medications known as triptans, such as Maxalt.

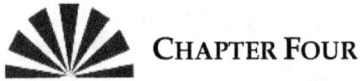 **CHAPTER FOUR**

# Fashions & Flashes & Home Décor

We all know what happens when we start the day in a slip- over sweater: By mid-morning we're wishing we had on a halter-top and shorts!  Since a hot flash is all about a massive and rapid release of body heat, it stands to reason that anything which stops that escape – such as a heavy or tightly knit sweater or jacket – is going to keep that flash going longer than it should. Sometimes it can even incite a second flash on the top of the first.

So, if you haven't already figured this out, this is not the time of life to load up on dresses with a long zipper up the back – no matter how great the sale is! It is, in fact, a time for dressing in layers.  This allows you to wear season-appropriate styles, but still do a little mini strip-tease without alarming co-workers, every time a flash comes on.

But this section isn't about the art of layered dressing - my guess is you've probably already figured that part out!  Instead I want to tell you a little bit about fabrics and the role they can play in not only keeping you more comfortable when you have a hot flash, but maybe even help you to reduce the number or intensity of the flashes you do have.

The key is to look for clothes in fabrics that don't hold in heat – fabrics that "breathe". This is important for two reasons.

First, a fabric that does "breathe" will allow body heat to escape more quickly – which means you won't feel as hot when you do have a flash.

But wearing cooler fabrics also helps moderate your body temperature, which in turn may help reduce the number of faulty brain-to-body signals able to  kick off a flash.

While this is important regarding the clothing and fabrics you wear during the day, it can be even more important when it comes to selecting both your sleep wear and your bedding.  Indeed, as any woman whose ever had to get up in the middle of the night to change a soaking wet nightgown can tell you, finding cool sleepwear is half the battle.  But I'm happy to tell you it's a battle you can win – both day & night.

## FABRICS TO LOOK FOR – AND AVOID

So what are fabrics that breathe? In the simplest terms they are the materials with a loose weave. In other words, when you tug on the fabric – or hold it up to the light – you can see tiny spaces between the threads. This is what ultimately will allow your body heat to escape – and so the fabric is said to "breathe".

Examples include most cotton, some polyester, mostly all polyester/cotton knits, wool, cashmere, linen, and almost any loosely woven fabric regardless of its content.

Fabrics that don't "breathe" are the ones that, when held up to the light, look dense – either there is no space between the fibers or they are so tightly woven it's difficult to see even light shine through them. Additionally, there are also certain man-made fibers – such as peachskin or other microfibers - that, regardless of their weave, make it hard for body heat to escape. According to *The Sewers Handbook*, by Bettie G. Roth and Chris Schultz, the fabrics most likely to hold in body heat include nylon, acetate, acrylic, modacrylic, many metallics, rayon, and some polyester fabrics.

Unfortunately, a lot of exercise clothing is made of nylon or combinations of nylon, polyester, and spandex, which can be exceedingly hot. And while exercise can ultimately help calm your hot flashes, (and you'll read more about how and why in Part II of this book) if you feel like your hair is on fire every time you work out you're less likely to do it. And who could blame you?

That's why it's very important to pay attention to the fabrics you're wearing not only when exercising, but also when doing any significant physical activity – even cleaning the house or power shopping in the mall!

If you stick to lighter weight fabrics that breathe – a cotton/polyester knit is great for working out – you'll be more comfortable, get more accomplished and I guarantee you'll have fewer hot flashes!

## NIGHT CLOTHES AND BEDDING: WHAT YOU NEED TO KNOW

If you think that most workout clothes have the potential to cause your body to overheat – and over flash – you're right. But it still pales in comparison to what simple, every day nighties and PJ's can do in terms of encouraging night sweats and sleep disruptions. As I'm sure you've already figured out, the vast majority of women's nightclothes are made of nylon, acrylic, or cotton – and all three can be a disaster if you suffer from night sweats.

The nylon and the acrylic hold in body heat – so you're going to be naturally warmer when you sleep. And that means your brain is likely to get the "cool down" message that triggers a hot flash a lot more often. As you read earlier, night sweats are, essentially hot flashes that occur while you sleep.

So, the more body heat your night clothes hold in, the more likely you are to wake up drenched in sweat. While cotton is a fabric that breathes, it's also one that holds moisture. And that means when hot flashes occur during sleep, all that extra perspiration has nowhere to go.

And that means you're just as likely to be awakened by the wetness as the heat. In fact, if you get a lot of hot flashes during your waking hours, you might also want to think twice about wearing all cotton, since a blend is less likely to leave you feeling damp.

Another "natural" fabric that breathes but may not be right for menopause, particularly in bedclothes, is silk. Not only does it also hold moisture, it can be very warm, particularly silk knit. If you want proof of that, just skim through any winter athletic-wear catalog. Most of the undergarments worn by skiers are made of silk knit - because it holds in body heat so well! The best fabrics for menopause nightclothes:

-Polyester-cotton blends, particularly soft knits.
-Polyester cotton woven blends
-Loosely woven or mesh cotton knits
-Mesh knits Fabrics with "wicking" ability that pull perspiration away from the body.

Many of these same fabric guidelines also apply to bedding, including sheets, pillowcases, and blankets. All three can contribute to night sweats by encouraging overheating, or keeping the heat you are generating from being easily dissipated in the air.

As such, be choosy when selecting your menopause bedding, opting for not only lighter covers than you might normally use during a particular season, but also choosing fabrics that "breathe."

Many women also report they are most comfortable with down blankets and comforters, even in summer. Indeed, one of the unique properties of down is that it works somewhat like an "adaptogen" - keeping the body heat at a more even temperature.

Do, however, be careful about the type of cover you use on your down blanket. If you wrap it in a fabric that doesn't breathe, you won't get the benefits of the down. Look for cotton/polyester blends or some loosely woven microfibers.

**Caution: Fabric Dye and Hot Flashes:** Whether choosing your nightclothes, day clothes, or bedding, be aware that certain fabric dyes can cause hot flashes in some women. It falls under the category of "allergic reaction", but during any other time in your life you might not even notice the connection. But when you're already prone to hot flushing, sometimes even a slight fabric dye allergy is enough to make a hot flash feel that much worse.

While most fabrics made in the US are properly rinsed so that dyes don't leave any irritating residues, the same is not true for many imported fabrics or garments made from imported fabric – particularly those sold by mass-market retailers. So if you find that you feel extra warm – or get more flashes – when you wear certain fabrics or colors, consider whether or not you could be having a reaction to the dye. Most often a few washings in cold water will get out the excess and make the item easier to tolerate.

## Wicking Night Clothes & Sheets

Over the past several years an entirely new category of "midlife" nightwear has made its way into the marketplace.

Known as "wick wear", it takes its cue from fabrics originally developed for athletes, particularly long distance runners, to help them stay cooler and dryer.

The principal behind "wickware" – also known as "thermo regulating fabric" – are polyester fibers that help "wick" or "pull" moisture from the surface of the skin and transfer it outside of the garment. It does so via nearly invisible micro-slits on the surface of the fabric, which work to rapidly absorb sweat from the surface of the skin and pull it away from the body and ultimately, to the outside of the fabric, where it quickly dries.

In fact, in many instances the fabric dries so quickly, it allows some women to completely avoid the sensation of "wetness" that frequently makes night sweats so uncomfortable.

So if you're a gal whose night sweats grow more intense – or more annoying – due to the feeling of being drenched in perspiration, then garments or sheets made with wicking technology will probably help you.

That said, while drier can mean cooler, it doesn't always – so don't be surprised if you still feel as warm as you did wearing regular nightwear or sleeping on regular sheets.

Also important to note: Some of these "wicking" fabrics can be quite stiff and hard and, as a friend of mine recently described it, "It felt like sleeping in one of those paper examining gowns!"

The warning here: Don't "go cheap" when searching out these garments or sheets – particularly if you are ordering on the Internet and can't see or feel what you are buying.

You can also look for products made with a newer wicking fabric called "CoolNew". It blends the typical polyester wicking fiber with a cotton fiber for a fabric that has the stay-dry properties with infinitely more softness to the touch.

Check our website YourMenpause.com for a listing of where to buy quality wickware sheets and nightclothes.

## DermaTherapy: Skin Care For Your Bed

One giant step up from traditional wicking bedding is a new technology known as Dermatherapy – nicknamed "Skin Care Bedding", and with good reason.

First, the specially developed micro fibers used in the fabric are ultra smooth to the touch. With no loose fibers to irritate dry, mid-life skin these sheets feel instantly softer to the touch.

But there's something more: These uniquely structured microfibers also work to distribute moisture evenly over the surface of the sheet. As that moisture evaporates, you don't get the usual "clammy" or "wet feeling" that can occur with cotton or even some cotton-poly fabrics.

The end result is a more comfortable sleep surface that is not only soft to the touch, but cooler and drier - no matter what your body is doing. Plus, an antimicrobial treatment means the sheets also feel and smell fresher – and there are fewer germs to cause skin irritation.

But you don't have to take my word for it: DermaTherapy is actually the first fabric that I know if that has been tested in a clinical trial - with specific, menopause-related sleep parameters in mind.

The research was conducted by Northeast Surgical Associates of Ohio, and involved 28 post menopausal women, all of whom had indicated quality of sleep issues, many related to night sweats and other menopause symptoms.

The study used two medically accepted evaluation tools to determine the women's sleep issues before and after using the DermaTherapy bedding. The first tool is   The Pittsburgh Sleep Quality Index (PSQI) - a questionnaire designed to assess sleep quality, sleep latency, sleep duration, habitual sleep efficiency, sleep disturbance, use of sleep medications and daytime dysfunction.

The second tool is a Quality of Life (QOL) assessment designed to measure an individual's ability to keep cool while sleeping, plus evaluate the amount of sweating and perceived comfort during a night's rest. At the start of the 8-week study nearly all the women participating had a sleep quality score of 9 – indicating they weren't sleeping well or comfortably.

After 8 weeks of sleeping on the DermaTherapy bedding the women were re-evaluated – and sleep scores took a dramatic jump.  Indeed, most of the women saw a significant improvement in sleep quality, and length of time they were able to comfortably sleep at night.  They also reported fewer disturbances – so they slept sounder. Interestingly, nearly all the women reported feeling better during the daytime with fewer menopause symptoms overall. Statistics also showed that quality of life improved substantially for most of the women, often within the first two weeks of using the DermaTherapy sheets.

During the remaining six weeks of the study the evaluation tools also determined the women had a higher level of uninterrupted sleep, and a greater ability to keep cooler and drier while sleeping, with the overall level of sweating reduced. As a bonus: The women also reported their skin actually felt better, with reduced dryness.

By the conclusion of the study, evaluation scores revealed that most of the women regained normal (pre-menopausal) sleep habits with the use of DermaTherapy bedding.

Currently the DermaTherapy technology is available for consumer purchase via a line of bedding known as "Cool Sensations." A queen-sized sheet set sells for about $45.00 and a set of pillowcases is about $40.00. For more information on the DermaTherapy products visit our website at www.YourMenopause.com

## MENOPAUSE PILLOWS & COOL RELIEF PRODUCTS

Whether you've been flashing for a while now, or you're just a few weeks into the "burn", you've no doubt heard about a variety of pillows purported to help reduce night sweats and, in some instances, even keep you cool during the day.

While some use a water-filled insert to create a pillow that remains cool while you sleep, others rely on various technologies to allow the pillow to pull heat from your head and disperse it so you don't feel as warm.

The goal, however, of all these products is to keep you cooler and more comfortable while you sleep.

But do they work? Again, much like sheets and other bedding items, a good deal of your satisfaction will depend on your expectations – and what you're looking for.

Moreover your own personal comfort level and the level and duration of your hot flashes will also make a difference when it comes to how satisfied you are with these products.

Indeed, for some women they can be a sleep saver that makes a huge difference; for others, after an hour or two the pillows provide only a minimal amount of cooling that makes almost no difference.

And because reactions can be so individual, it's difficult to make any universal recommendations.

But what I can do is clue you in on how some of the most popular menopause pillows and mattress pads work – and what, if any, medical studies show about how well they can keep you cool.

# The Menopause Pillow:
# Some Popular Options

### Product: The Chillow
Approximate Cost: $30.00 - $40.00
Size: 21"L -- 13.5"W -- approx 1/2" D with water added
Weight: About 5.5 pounds filled.

**What It Is:** Although it was one of the first, and arguably remains one of the most popular in the "menopause" pillow category, the Chillow is not actually a pillow. Instead, it's an insert that combines a highly porous memory foam cover with a medical grade non-toxic vinyl insert, and a   flocked material on the back to help it "grip" to your pillow. You fill the Chillow with about 3.5 pints of tap water - which the foam absorbs- and  then use the vacuum sealer to pull out all the air. You slip the Chillow insert between your pillowcase and your actual pillow – or lie on it directly.

Additional versions: **The Pink Sweet Relief Chillow** – about half the size as a traditional Chillow and weighs about 3 pounds.

**The Promise:** Using a proprietary technology known as "SmoothSoft" a Chillow is said to combine certain properties of thermodynamics (the science of heat and energy) to pull warmth from your head and release it into the air.

This continual releasing of heat allows the Chillow insert to remain cool to the touch at all times.

**The Reality:** If you're looking for the icy-cold feel of a snowball against your skin, this isn't it. In fact, even the maker of The Chillow asserts that the goal of the insert is not to remain super cool *all the time,* but rather to react with your body temperature, cooling you down only when you need it. So, at the start of the night, when your metabolism is still revved from a day of activity, your head will be hotter- and the Chillow will be cooler. As you approach morning, however, and your body temperature has naturally cooled during the night, the Chillow will be substantially less cool to the touch.

That said, if, somewhere around dawn, you heat up with a night sweat, the Chillow is not going to suddenly get cold again. So in this respect, its usefulness may be best allocated to those who need the most cooling when they fall asleep.

You can also make the Chillow feel quite a bit cooler if you put it in the refrigerator (not the freezer!) for up to 20 minutes. While this will make it initially feel cooler to the touch, it won't do much to keep it cooler through the night.

For many women, the solution is to simply purchase two or more Chillows and interchange them during the night as they start to get warmer. However, if you're someone who has trouble falling back asleep, this might not be the system the works for you.

**The Chillow Plus:** As the latest addition to the Chillow line, this version does away with the flocked backing and replaces it with a smooth membrane-like material that allows it to stay cool on both sides of the insert. This can be a plus since oftentimes all you need to do to feel a cooler sensation is flip the pillow over. That gives you a cooler sleep surface.

The Chillow Plus also uses higher quality foam and it holds more water (up to 80 ounces) than the standard Chillow, so it is said to stay cooler longer . Some say it's also softer to the touch. One caveat: It does weigh substantially more (depending on how much water fill you include). It retails for around $ 50.00.

Other versions include the Sweet Petite and the Mini-Chillow. Both are smaller in size (14" x 10" x 5") and they weigh less – about 3 pounds. Both these smaller versions do have the same double-sided cooling membrane.

PRODUCT: IsoCool™
Approximate Cost: $25-$29.00
Size: Standard, Queen, King, 3" thick.
Weight: 3 to 4 pounds depending on size

What It Is: IsoCool™ pillows (mattress toppers also available) feature Outlast® Adaptive Comfort® material – a type of filling that adjusts to the body's changing temperature. Tiny microscopic beads inside the pillow sense the body's temperature and respond accordingly.

The Promise: Because this pillow acts as a kind of temperature sensor, if you're too warm the pillow absorbs heat so you feel cooler; if you're cold, it releases heat and feels warm to the touch. Since IsoCool™ products feature the highest available concentration of micro beads, they claim to be the most effective in this category of pillows – as well as the most comfortable. The pillows are also available in two luxurious and supportive fills: One type is made from a spiral-spun polyester, the other, from Viscose-elastic foam. The IsoCool™ mattress topper is available as a polyester cover or as a 3-inch, high-density Visco-elastic foam mattress pad with a polyester cover.

**The Reality:** I tried the foam version of this pillow and found that it did feel cool to the touch. That said, it did warm up relatively quickly – still cooler than most foam pillows but definitely warmer than when I first laid down. So, while it is definitely cooler than most foam pillows, if you're looking for an icy blast in the middle of a blazing flash or night sweat, this probably isn't the pillow for you.

I also found that this version of the pillow had a very strong "foam" odor. So, if you're sensitive to these kinds of smells, opt for the spiral spun polyester version instead.

**PRODUCT: HOT FLASH FRIDGE PILLOW**
Approximate Cost: $9.95
Weight – About 4 pounds fully inflated
Size: 11 x 9

**What It Is:** Based on the neck wraps that used to cool outdoor workers in summer, these ingenuous pillows are filled with water absorbing crystals that stay cool for days – even in hot temperatures.

**The Promise:** These pillows are designed to feel cool even after you are burning up! And while they arrive flat, weighing only a few ounces, once soaked in water, they grow cold and inflate to about 6 inches thick. The outside fabric dries super quickly – and if you wipe it off with a towel it's dry in less than one minute. But because it's the crystals inside that absorb the water and hold it, the pillow stays constantly cool. For an extra punch of icy coolness, you can refrigerate the inflated pillow for about a half hour.

**The Reality:** This pillow works! And it works better than anything I've tried in this category. Moreover, considering that it's filled with crystals, it's not hard at all – about equal to a very firm pillow. I've also found that if you soak it for less time, it doesn't inflate as much – and you can easily slip it on top of another pillow – so you get the coolness next to your skin with the comfort of your regular pillow underneath.

The one caveat: You can't wash these pillows with any kind of soap. If soap comes in contact with the crystals (and it can permeate the fabric) it can lead to a skin irritation. But if you simply place it in a pillow case, you shouldn't have any problems keeping it clean.

There is a also a smaller "headache" pillow version, 4"x6" in size. I usually soak it in water then slip it into a zip loc baggy and then into my purse – for an instant cooling sensation any time I need it!

Both pillows are available online at:
Shop.CoolCollars.net/main.sc or visit
YourMenopause.com for more information.

## MORE HOT FLASH BEDROOM ADVICE

It stands to reason that when you're in a hot environment, a hot flash is going to feel worse. And you probably already know that any room that is hot *and* stuffy can actually "trip" your temperature sensors and bring a hot flash on.

But what you might not realize is that extreme temperature *changes,* such as going from a cool air conditioned room into the broiling sun, or going from very cold icy temperatures into a very warm house, office or store, can also trigger a hot flash and have you burning up in no time flat.

For this reason one of the best ways to minimize hot flashes during the day to is keep your home at a moderate and even temperature. This will help minimize changes from one room to the next, or when going from indoors to outdoors.

In terms of night sweats, it's likely you will feel a lot better if you can keep your sleeping environment as cool as possible. If you have air conditioning, use it in summer months, but you don't have to turn to "arctic" to get the best relief. In fact, super cold temperatures may actually interfere with sleep.

Instead, keeping the temperature between 66 and 68 degrees should be the most comfortable for sleeping. In fall and winter months, always leave the window open just a crack, to allow some cool air to mingle with the hot air from your radiators, and help keep your bedroom a more moderate temperature.

Of course sometimes there is simply nothing we can do about the ambient temperature of a room – particularly when it's not our house!  If you're visiting a friend for the weekend, for example, or when you're at a dinner party, in your office, at a school function with your kids, at the mall shopping – in fact almost anyplace outside of your own home it can be difficult to control the temperature.

One solution is to always keep a glass of ice water or a can of cold soda handy – but don't drink it. Instead, press it against the inside of your wrist when you feel a flash coming on – and it might just short circuit the temperature changes enough to keep the flash at bay.

If you know you're going to be in a warm environment, you can also prepare ahead by investing in a small, insulated bag – the kind used to carry medications that are heat sensitive. One such product is called the Icy Bag – and it comes with a small gel insert that you freeze. Once inserted in the bag, it stays cold for up to 8 hours.  When you feel a flush coming on you can slip the gel insert out of the bag, and  press it either against your wrist or the inside of your elbow, or hold it on the back of your neck. In some instances it can stop a flash – other times it can help reduce the intensity and help you get through it quicker and easier.  It retails for $19.99.

Another similar option is called the "Glisten Pad".  It features a cooling, ice-blue non toxic gel pad, (the kind used by physical therapists to treat muscular inflammation), which fits nicely into a soft, ultra absorbent micro fiber pouch, and then, an insulated zippered carry case.

To use the Glisten Pad simply chill the gel insert in the refrigerator for 30 minutes, slip it into the plushy microfiber pouch and it's ready to be applied to your skin for instant "cool flash" relief. If you are already perspiring, the micro fiber quickly absorbs the moisture and wicks it away from your skin.

The insulated bag is designed to keep the Glisten Pad cool for as long as possible. It sells for $19.99 online.

For outdoor activities and sport events, nothing beats the "Cool Thing" a neck wrap filled with moisture-retaining beads. You soak the wrap in cold water, wipe the outside covering dry, and toss it in your handbag. When you get warm, slip it around your neck and voila! Hot flash gone! "Cool Thing" stays cold for up to 12 hours – and to refresh it all you need is cold tap water! Other versions are known as "Cool Collars" or "Cooling Scarves" and are available on line at several different websites. You can learn more about all these products at YourMenopause.com.

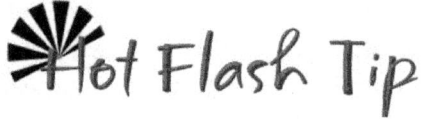

## Hot Flash Tip

In studies of women using the anti-cancer drug Tamoxifen, 400 units of vitamin E daily reduced the incidence of hot flashes by a significant margin. You can also add more vitamin E rich foods to your diet, especially nuts. But be careful not to over indulge – nuts can be high in calories.

**CHAPTER FIVE**

# The Hot Flash Solution

# Lifestyle Diary

Now that you have a better idea of not only how and why your hot flashes and night sweats occur, but also some of the lifestyle factors can bring them on, it's time to see how all this information fits into your personal hot flash profile.

The program designed to help you do just that is **The Hot Flash Solution Lifestyle Diary**. In essence, it's a simple way of keeping track of your flashes, the factors that can trigger them, and how the two relate.

While the categories are the same for all women – such as food, clothing, activities, etc. - the individual listings within each category will be *very specific to you*. To use the *Lifestyle Diary*, you'll enter the time of your hot flash in the column on the far left side of the page, and then follow across the chart from left to right, where you will find a series of boxes, each one marked with an icon, and each icon representing a specific lifestyle factor. Your goal: To fill in the boxes under any icon that applies, each time a flash occurs.

For example, under the clothing icon you might enter *pink wool sweater*; under the food icon you might enter *chocolate bar*; under the beverage icon, *iced tea*. The point is to notate as many factors as you can related to each flash you have – and to be as specific as you can. This is particularly important in the food and drink sections. Don't, for example, write "ate lunch" or "had a drink".

Instead write down what you ate and what you drank for lunch. And if you had a alcoholic drink note if it was wine, beer, whiskey, a mixed drink, etc. Again, the more specific you can be the easier it will be to interpret your chart and zero in on your hot flash triggers.

And while sometimes you may have every box filled in across an entire row, other times you may only have one or two boxes filled in.

Each chart has a space for 7 flashes – the average number most women have in a day.

However, if you have more, feel free to print out more than one chart page for each day; if you have fewer flashes, then use one sheet for several days.

After you have completed 7 –14 pages of entries – equal to 1 to 2 weeks worth of hot flashes – it's time to sit down analyze your results. And I promise it will be an exciting eye opener! In fact, don't be surprised if you discover reasons behind your hot flashes you never would have guessed!

## WHAT TO LOOK FOR

The main objective with the **The Hot Flash Solutions Diary is** to help you uncover *hot flash trigger patterns.* Essentially, these are boxes that "match up" from flash to flash.

Sometimes the pattern will be obvious right away – like recognizing that a hot flash always seems to arrive right after eating a chocolate bar, or drinking a cup of coffee. Other times it may take a little detective work to find the common thread. For example, under your clothing icon boxes you might have filled out "red sweater, "green blouse", and "bathrobe" – which don't seem to be related. But a closer look could tell you if they are all made of the same fabric, or one of the fabrics listed in the fashion chapter as holding in body heat.

If you don't begin to see patterns emerge within the first week, not to worry. For some women it can take two to three weeks to find the common threads. This can be the case if your life is full and you are less of a creature of habit, or when lifestyle factors are triggering a smaller percentage of your flashes. Either way, if you have some patience, within a month or less I promise you will have a much better idea of what's contributing to your flashes and night sweats, and the lifestyle factors playing the biggest role.

Once you do, you can use both the lifestyle advice in Part One this book, and the natural treatment options in Part Two to create a truly *personal* Hot Flash Solution for you!

To help you better understand the Lifestyle Diary chart – and make it more fun to use - I created icons for each of the entries.

What follows are definitions for each icon – what each category should include. While you don't have to memorize the various categories it is a good idea to at least familiarize yourself with each one. Then, when you feel a hot flash coming on you'll know what you need to think about – and what factors you need to note as true for you.

You can also print out the icon definitions and the chart at TheHotFlashSolution.com.

IMPORTANT TO NOTE: Remember, not all of these factors will be linked to every hot flash you have. And, in fact, some of them may not apply to you at all, during *any hot flash*. Other times some factors may be present, while others aren't. Moreover, you may find various sub topics within each category that are more personal to you.

The point to remember is that you are looking to establish a *pattern of factors* that are present during the majority of *your* hot flashes. Once you identify that pattern, you have taken the first step towards identifying your personal hot flash triggers. Once you do, you can work on eliminating or reducing those triggers – and in the process you'll see just how easy it can be to take control of your hot flashes and night sweats for good!

HOT FLASH LIFESTYLE DIARY ICON DEFINITIONS

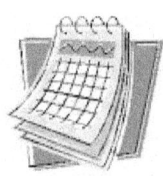

**Date And Time**
In order to calculate your hot flash triggers it's important to know the date and time they occurred. You don't have to be pin-point accurate – it's okay to say "afternoon", or "morning", but if you do know the time, enter it here. Ultimately, the more detailed your information, the easier it will be to pinpoint your triggers.

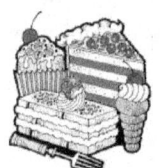

**What did I eat?**
In this box list everything you ate in the 15 to 30 minutes before your hot flash occurred. You can list general categories – like candy, ice cream, cake, a hamburger, a bag of chips. Or you can be more specific such as chocolate candy, vanilla cake, or strawberry ice cream. Also important: Note the temperature of the food – was it cold like ice cream, warm like soup, or room temperature like cake? The more specific you can be, the easier it will be to track down your hot flash trigger.

**What did I drink?**

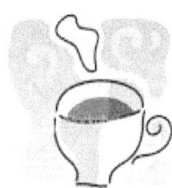

This box should contain all non-alcoholic drinks you consumed in the 10 to 30 minutes prior to your hot flash. Categories include coffee, tea, hot chocolate, soda, juice, ice water, iced tea, iced coffee, mocha latte. The more specific you can be the easier it will be to track your hot flash trigger. *Very important:* Note whether the beverage was hot or cold.

## What I Am Wearing

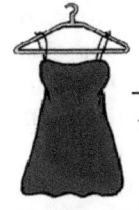 This not only refers to the article of clothing – such as a sweater or bathrobe – but more important, the fabric you are wearing, such as cotton, spandex, nylon, flannel, polyester, etc. If you don't know what kind of fabric you are wearing, then identify the article of clothing – such as "pink long sleeve shirt", or "white sweater". As long as you know what the item is, it can help you to identify if it may be a trigger. If you do establish that what you wear triggers a hot flash, you can back track and see what all the items have in common. Often it will be the fabric, or the color – an indication of the dye.

### What I Am Doing Right Now?

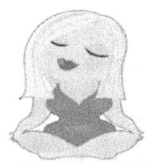 Are you exercising? Vacuuming? Doing laundry? Having sex? Smoking? Thinking about having sex? ☺ Meditating? Watching television? Cooking? Eating? At your computer? Talking on the phone? Taking a bath? Driving? Whatever activity you are engaged in at the time your flash occurs - *write it down*. You don't have to stop and do it that minute – but try to remember what you were doing when your flash occurred, and fill it in when you can.

### What Am I Feeling?

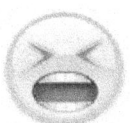 Happy? Sad? Aggravated? Stressed? Furious? Sleepy? Hurt? Upset? Contented? Relaxed? Frightened? Turned On? Anxious? Depressed? Whatever you're feeling when the flash strikes, jot it down – you don't need a lot of details, just an indication of how you were feeling when the flash hit.

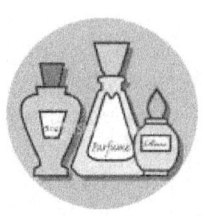

**What Am I Smelling?** From the scent of your favorite perfume, to the laundry detergent you just dumped into the washer, the fumes from the office copy machine, your dish washing detergent, shower gel, shampoo, your best friends new carpet, the oven as it self-cleans, your co-workers perfume, new cut grass, a bouquet of flowers - if there is an obvious fragrance present at the time you are getting a hot flash, enter it here.

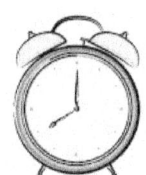

**Activity: The Last 30 Minutes**
Different from *"What Am I Doing Now?"* this is a record of what you were doing in *the 30 minutes or so before your flash hit.* This is also the place where you enter the relative temperature of the room *before your flash hit.* Was it cold, warm, just right? Also note if any temperature change occurred – hot to cold, or cold to hot, as you came in or went out.

**Alcohol Consumption :** For some women alcohol brings on an immediate hot flash, for others the reaction is delayed or linked to the total amount consumed over a period of hours. For still others, it's

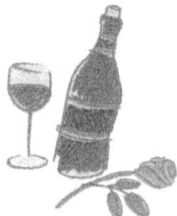

the type of alcohol that becomes the trigger. So try to be as specific as you can when filling in this section - noting the type of alcohol, and the amount – such as 2nd glass of the day.

Download a larger version of this chart at:
www.TheHotFlashSolution.com

Today's Date:_____ Date of Last Menstrual Cycle_____ Hot Flash Diary Lifestyle Chart

| | | | | | | | | |
|---|---|---|---|---|---|---|---|---|
| Time of Flash: | | | | | | | | |
| Time of Flash: | | | | | | | | |
| Time of Flash: | | | | | | | | |
| Time of Flash: | | | | | | | | |
| Time of Flash: | | | | | | | | |
| Time of Flash: | | | | | | | | |
| Time of Flash: | | | | | | | | |
| Time of Flash: | | | | | | | | |

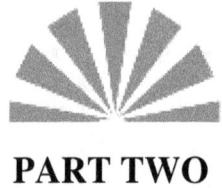

# PART TWO

# The Safe
# Natural Treatments
# That Can
# Change Your Life

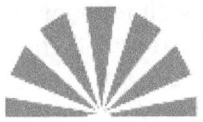

# Introduction: Part Two

For many of you reading this book, simply identifying your personal hot flash triggers, and making small but significant lifestyle changes, may be all that's necessary to get your hot flashes and night sweats under complete control.

While they may not vanish completely, they can certainly decrease in frequency and intensity to the point where they no longer impinge on your life or lifestyle.

For others, however, problems may still persist.But the good news here: If you do need more help, there are a variety of safe natural treatments available. What's more, conquering your personal hot flash triggers will clear the way for most of them to work better and more efficiently! And that is precisely what you will find in part two of this book: The all-natural treatments that can really make a difference.

Based on solid medical research and published clinical trials, I've pulled together the best and the safest most natural, easiest solutions capable of making a difference in how you feel.

Certainly not every treatment is right for every woman. Some may work amazingly well for some – and not at all for others. That's also part of your personal hot flash profile.

But I can promise you that you will find something in this next section that can and will help you. Also remember, if you try one or two treatments and they *don't work* – please don't give up, and do go on to try more. It is very likely that you will find at least one, or a combination of several remedies, that will make a significant difference in how you feel.

Moreover, I also urge you to give the treatments time to work. While some can yield results in two weeks, most take from 12 to 16 weeks to see the full result, so have patience!

By identifying your personal hot flash triggers and trying the solutions found in this section, you will have the best one-two punch available to knock out hot flashes and put night sweats to rest for good!

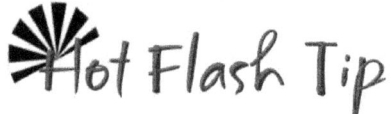

You can quickly stop a hot flash – or reduce the
impact - by running your wrists under cold
water. Don't have a faucet nearby?
Then just press the inside of your wrist against a
glass of ice water or a cold can of soda.
For even faster relief, press the can to the inside
of your elbow. All three actions will help reset
your body's thermostat and help your hot flash
to cool down fast!

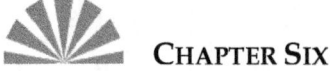 **CHAPTER SIX**

# The Hot Flash Diet: Eat & Feel Better!

It's no secret that food – and specifically good nutrition – can have an enormous impact on our health. In fact, in the past decade we have learned more about links between good food and good health than we ever imagined possible.

And, I'm happy to tell you that at least some of those links connect directly to what you eat during menopause.

Not only will certain foods give you a nutritional boost that can set the stage for a happier, healthier "second act", but there is some evidence to show they can also impact hot flashes.

You already read how certain foods can make hot flashes worse – including spicy dishes, too much sugar, caffeine and alcohol. But now you'll discover which foods can actually have a positive impact on hot flashes and night sweats, helping you feel better and helping you gain important control over many menopause symptoms.

## THE SOY SOLUTION

Among the most promising "kitchen" treatments for hot flashes are soybeans. Whether taken as a supplement or as a food, there is significant clinical evidence to show soy can and does have an impact on menopause symptoms, particularly hot flashes.

This natural power comes from the fact that soy is considered a "phytoestrogen" – a source of estrogen that comes from plants, and it is very similar to what is produced in a woman's body. (See Chapter 10 for more on natural hormones).

In fact, all plants manufacture a form of estrogen, which they need to survive and grow. In many instances these "phytoestrogens" are remarkably similar to *estriol* – a type of estrogen produced in a woman's body – but just in a weaker concentration.

Nonetheless, many phytoestrogens have at least some ability to function like a natural hormone, particularly in regard to "estrogen receptors". Remember, these are the areas of the body where estrogen normally settles, influencing the way our body functions, and ultimately the way we feel.

As you read earlier, estrogen helps control the temperature circuitry of the hypothalamus. So, when levels become unstable, that circuitry no longer works properly – and hot flashes can occur. Many believe that "phytoestrogens" can help fill in that gap, offering enough estrogen-like activity to keep the circuitry in good working order and in the process control hot flashes.

Of course one way to get phytoestrogens is through natural hormone therapy. And you'll learn more about the pros and cons of that later in this book.

But another way is through foods high in phytoestrogens. Although available from a number of plants, the most studied and some say the most effective forms are found in soybeans. For many women, simply adding more soy to their daily diet is enough of a hormone boost to reduce symptoms.

## HOW SOY CONTROLS HOT FLASHES

Soy plants contain three of the most potent forms of phytoestrogen available. They include genistein, daidzein and glycitein. Collectively they fall under a category known as "isoflavone".

A second, slightly different class of phytoestrogens is known as "lignans, found in foods such as flax seed and some legumes. (And you'll learn more about these in a few minutes).

Together, isoflavones and lignans comprise one of the most-studied of all natural menopause treatment options. Here's a sampling of that research.

- In one 16-week study of 75 women published in the journal *Menopause* in 2000, nearly 61% of those experiencing at least 7 hot flashes a day found relief with daily use of a soy extract containing 70mg of genistein and

70mg of daidzein. This was compared to just 21% in the group who took a placebo pill.

- In a second, larger study, also published in *Menopause* the same year, 177 women with 5 or more hot flashes daily took an isoflavone extract of 50mg of genistein and 50mg of daidzein daily. In just 12 weeks they saw dramatic improvement. More importantly, ultra sound examinations showed no thickening of their uterine lining – a potential problem with traditional HRT.

- A third 6-week study involved 51 women with hot flashes who compared a diet containing 20mg of soy protein daily (34 mg of isoflavones) to a diet high in complex carbohydrates. The results, also published in the journal *Menopause,* found the group eating the soy had a significant reduction in hot flashes, while the group eating the diet high in complex carbohydrates experienced little change. Those who split their soy into two meals saw the greatest decrease in symptoms.

And this, it seems was only the beginning.

As time passed, more and more studies began to validate the impact of soy on not only hot flashes, but many menopause symptoms – and consequences of the menopause years.

For example, studies in the *New England Journal of Medicine* and other top journals reported that soy has the power to lower cholesterol and blood pressure, as well as decrease the risk of stroke-related blood clots.

In one study featured in the *Journal of Clinical Nutrition*, just 40 mg of soy protein daily had a significant impact on lumbar bone density, helping to protect women from the bone thinning effects of osteoporosis.

In another major study of some 5,000 Japanese women, researchers found that women who ate soy on a regular basis were healthier overall – and had the fewest menopause symptoms.

The very latest research, published in the journal CANCER in August of 2008 found that the isoflavone compounds in soy, as well as in tea, appeared to reduce the risk of ovarian cancer by as much as 49%.
But that's not all. In fact, even with the far more common incidence of breast cancer, doctors are finding soy may help reduce risks.

In one brand new 15 year study of more than 35,000 women researchers found that consuming as little as 10.6 mg of soy daily could reduce the risk of breast cancer by nearly 20%.

Continue to eat that portion size over a ten year period and watch your risk of breast cancer decrease by a whopping 64%. The research was conducted by the National University of Singapore and presented at a breast cancer symposium in August 2008.

## A WORD OF CAUTION ABOUT SOY

There is indeed, an overwhelming amount of evidence to support the goodness of soy, particularly in menopause-aged women. That said, there are some studies that question a "soy overload", citing that *too much of a good thing* is, well, a bad thing. In one laboratory study phytoestrogens added to breast cancer cells in a lab dish made those cells grow at an alarming rate, responding much the way they would if flooded with estrogen. So, while eating soy in moderation may lower your risk of breast cancer, eating too much might increase your risk.

This may be particularly important to consider if you have a personal or family history of breast cancer. If this is the case, then definitely speak with your doctor before adding soy to your diet in any significant quantities.

Additionally, there is some preliminary data showing that some forms of soy – particularly tofu - may have a detrimental effect on memory, and could encourage some forms of dementia.

While the research has been primarily on men - and it's still a long way off from being validated as a general health recommendation - if you do have a personal or family history of early dementia or Alzheimer's disease, you may also want to limit your consumption of tofu, or balance it with nutrients known to be useful in these conditions, particularly folic acid and other B vitamins.

GETTING THE MOST FROM YOUR SOY

If you decide to add soy into your diet, it's important to recognize that not all soy foods are equally rich in the important "isoflavone" compound.

Moreover, even in those foods which contain the

primary menopause isoflavones - daidzein and genistein - it's important that also they be present in the proper ratio. The best way to insure this, is to derive your soy intake from natural foods.

Generally speaking, raw soybeans contain between 2mg and 4mg of isoflavones per gram. Popular soy foods such as tofu, soymilk or miso contain about 30 to 40 mg of isoflavone per serving, usually in the proper ratio.

If you choose 60 grams of roasted soybeans, or 75 grams of green soybeans you'll end up with a whopping 100 mg of isoflavone!

Textured vegetable protein is another popular source of soy, often found in many soy burgers. You'll need about 70 grams per serving to reach your goal.

If you're baking with soy flour, you'll get about 50mg of isoflavone with every half cup you use. Divide that by the number of servings your recipe yields and you'll see how much you'll need to eat to meet your soy intake goal.

**Soy Foods To Avoid:** Packaged products made from soy protein concentrates are not usually a reliable source of the proper soy menopause nutrients. They frequently show up in products like frozen soy burgers or snack bars, and can fool you into believing you're getting more bang for your soy buck than you actually are. While some of these products do contain adequate amounts of isoflavone, depending on how they were processed, many do not.

How to tell? Read the label! It should state the complete nutritional content. If it doesn't, contact the company either online or by mail.

You should also avoid what is known as "second generation" soy products – items that boast the use of soy on the label, but don't really contain enough of it to make any real dietary difference. Again, the label is your best guide.

## THE POWER OF FLAX SEED

If soy is not one of your favorite foods, take heart, you're not alone. For some women it can cause excess gas, while others simply find they don't like the taste. If this is the case for you, then look to foods that contain "lignans" - another good plant source of phytoestrogen.

Derived from the outer portion of certain fibrous plants this compound is also believed to mimic the effects of estrogen in the body. Although there is less research attesting to the effectiveness than there is for soy, there is clearly some evidence that its hormone-balancing effects are similar.

Plus, it can also offer some additional antioxidant and anti inflammatory activity thanks to compounds known as omega 3 fatty acids, which are also present. Among the most potent sources of lignans is ground flax seed meal, but flax seed oil (available in capsules) can also provide some of the benefits. Indeed, not only does flax have the ability to act like an estrogen, ameliorating hot flashes and night sweats, studies have shown it also has anti-cancer effects. In one study just two teaspoons of flax oil daily helped to reduce tumor growth in both breast and colon cancer patients.

Currently flaxseed is also being studied as a way of reducing cholesterol. Since a drop in estrogen can often lead to an increase in blood cholesterol levels, it may be an especially important food to eat during this time of life – not only for its ability to impact hot flashes, but also for the effects on your overall health. Moreover, flax is also packed with a particular type of omega 3 fatty acid known as alphalinolenic acid. This has anti-inflammatory properties that may have a positive impact on blood vessels and even decrease your risk of heart attack.

Because, however, flax seed can hard for some women to digest – and some may even be highly allergic – it's a good idea to start with a very low quantity. According to nutritionist Elaine Magee, RD, you should begin with as little as ¼ teaspoon a day, and if you don't experience a bad reaction, increase the amount gradually –  up to 1 teaspoon a few times a week.

IMPORTANT: You must either grind the flax seeds, or buy them already ground, since eating the whole seeds will cause them to pass through your system undigested.

You can mix ground flax seed into any number of recipes, including muffins, bread, cookies, or use it in smoothies.  For some recipes that include flax seed visit www.YourMenopause.com.

## FRUITS & VEGETABLES
## WITH AN ESTROGEN TWIST

I know…this sounds like a new cocktail recipe from *"Sex In The City – The Senior Years"*! But in reality, I'm referring to fruits and vegetables that contain both phytoestrogens – the plant estrogens you just read about – as well as a concentrated amount of the mineral boron. That's the "estrogen twist".

What's the connection to hot flashes? According to Magee boron helps the body hold on to estrogen – so eating fruits and vegetables high in both boron and phytoestrogens will offer you a higher level of hormonal support. And that could mean you not only feel better during menopause, but you might have fewer hot flashes as well.

Moreover, since boron is also an important mineral for bone health, it offers some protection against osteoporosis, the bone thinning disorder that can zap your skeletal strength and increase your risk of bone breaks as you age.

Indeed, one of the reasons osteoporosis strikes women after menopause has to do with the loss of estrogen. Since estrogen helps keep calcium in bones, anything you can do to supplement the process after estrogen levels start to drop can have an important impact on your bone health.

You can also increase bone health by getting up to 20 minutes of sun exposure a day. Sunlight helps our body make vitamin D – and it is this nutrient that helps bring calcium into our bones. While too much sun exposure can increase your risk of skin cancer and skin aging, a little can go a long way in protecting your bones. What can also help: Taking a supplement with up to 1,000 mg of vitamin D daily.

To ensure you are getting both phytoestrogens and boron, try the following fruits and vegetables – which have the highest content of both!

### Fruits :
✓ Plums
✓ Prunes
✓ Strawberries
✓ Apples
✓ Tomatoes
✓ Pears
✓ Grapes
✓ Oranges
✓ Red Raspberries.

### Vegetables:
✓ Asparagus
✓ Beets
✓ Bell Peppers
✓ Broccoli stem
✓ Cabbage
✓ Cauliflower
✓ Carrots
✓ Cucumbers
✓ Lettuce
✓ Onions
✓ Soybeans
✓ Sweet Potatoes
✓ Turnips.

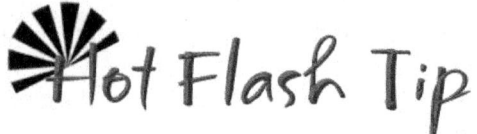 Hot Flash Tip

Do you find that your hot flashes come on more quickly just after you've put on your make-up? If so look to your foundation as one possible culprit!

Some women have reported that long lasting foundations, as well as foundations containing chemical sunscreens can bring on a hot flash. If this seems true for you, cut out your foundation for a day or two and see if makes a difference. If so, try switching to a moisturizing, calming foundation – such as those by Clinique or Prescriptives.

You can also try putting on a make-up primer first. This puts a layer between your skin and the foundation that may help reduce facial flushing. A great dual-action primer and moisturizer is Garnier Ultra Lift Serum.
As a bonus: It's also cooling and calming to the skin!

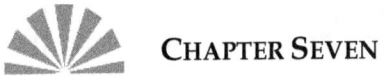 **CHAPTER SEVEN**

# Mother Nature's Garden: Herbs to Cool You Down!

Among the most popular approaches to do-it-yourself hot flash therapy is the use of herbal compounds. These are supplements derived from natural plant substances, some of which come with a long history of providing relief.

Indeed, the German E Commission – a government organization similar to the United States FDA (Food and Drug Administration) - has been championing the use of certain herbal substances for the treatment of menopause symptoms for over 40 years.

At the same time, there are lots of "sham" herbal treatments making the rounds – products that tempt us with enticing ads and promises of instant hot flash relief – but in the end, rarely deliver.

To help you sort through the hype and find those ingredients that hold the most promise, I've combed the medical journals and the clinical trials to find out exactly which of these products have been tested and what those tests found, in terms of not only effectiveness, but also safety.

And, I'm happy to report that I have found several formulations and ingredients that do hold important promise for relief. While not all herbal supplements will work equally well for all women – even the ones with a good clinical record of success – at the very least you can use this information to narrow down the odds, so that whatever product you decide to try will at least have some record of success.

Of course, it goes without saying that symptoms should always be verified by your doctor and you must let her know if you decide to take any herbal supplements of any kind, particularly if you are already using other medication on a regular or semi regular basis.

Remember, any herb that is strong enough to help you is strong enough to cause you harm – so approach use with the same caution you would when considerin any prescription drug.

## BLACK COHOSH – THE HOT FLASH HERB

With a history of use that dates back more than 100 years in the United States, and longer than that within the American Indian culture, black cohosh is indeed one of the most utilized, as well as one of the well-studied herbs in use today. Traditionally it was used to treat a variety of "female" ailments, including menstrual pain and labor pain, for which American Indian women boiled the roots and drank the liquid. It was, in fact, believed to be so effective that between 1890 and 1926 the US government officially listed black cohosh as a "drug".

More recently, black cohosh has become a mainstay menopause treatment for the European community. For the past 40 years more than 1.5 million women have used black cohosh as a treatment for menopause symptoms, particularly hot flashes. And it's approved by the German E Commission for this purpose, in doses ranging from 40 mg to 200 mg daily.

Perhaps most importantly, since 1982 there have been dozens of clinical trials offering important evidence that this herb is helpful in treating not only hot flashes but other symptoms of perimenopause as well, including anxiety, sweating, insomnia, even the shrinkage of vaginal tissue which often leads to uncomfortable or painful sex during this time of life.

## HOW AND WHY BLACK COHOSH WORKS

The essential compound found within the black cohosh plant is a substance known as "triterpene," a natural chemical that some research shows may have estrogen-like effects. In this respect it is believed to help balance the otherwise unstable estrogen levels linked to hot flashes.

Other research suggests the success of black cohosh may be related to its impact on the hypothalamus gland. Remember, this is the part of the brain linked to temperature control and also the circuitry involved in hot flashes. According to preventive medicine expert Dr. Jan MacBarron from Atlanta, Georgia, black cohosh appears to work directly on the hypothalamus gland, acting much like estrogen to prevent those false "brain-to-body" temperature signals that initiate a hot flash. In this respect black cohosh may reduce or even eliminate hot flashes.

And, in fact, a brand new study just published by researchers from the University of Michigan has offered more evidence this is the case. Their study was the first to use sophisticated brain imaging techniques to actually prove that black cohosh not only enters the temperature pathways in the brain, but once there is accepted in much the same way that estrogen is – in many of the same areas.

What is perhaps most interesting about black cohosh is that it appears to work as an "adaptogen" - a compound capable of acting different ways depending on what the body needs. For example, in women whose estrogen levels are low, black cohosh appears to support those functions that require estrogen.

At the same time if hormone levels are too high, black cohosh then acts like an anti-estrogen. In fact, studies have shown that, when used regularly for 6 months or less, black cohosh stops hot flashes without increasing health risks associated with an estrogen overload – such as breast or endometrial cancer.

Moreover laboratory tests have shown that when used for 6 months or less black cohosh has no negative impact on breast cancer cells – a medical fact that has led some experts to conclude this herb may be safe even for women who have a history of estrogen-sensitive conditions, including not only breast cancer but also abnormal cell growth within the uterus, or even a history of endometriosis, polyps or fibroid tumors.

In fact, in one study conducted by experts from the University Of Pennsylvania School Of Medicine and published in the *International Journal of Cancer*, 17 different types of natural treatments for menopause symptoms were compared. The result: Only one, a black cohosh remedy that sells by the brand name Remifemin, appeared to actually reduce the risk of breast cancer by up to 60%.

Of course every woman's health history is unique so if you are at risk for breast cancer, or have any of these other hormone-related conditions in your family or personal health history, do check with your doctor before using black cohosh or any herbal treatment. And if you try this or any herb and your symptoms worsen, or you experience any other significant problems, stop, and talk to your doctor.

## FINDING THE RIGHT BLACK COHOSH

Certainly, there is adequate evidence that black cohosh works – at least for some women. One study published in the journal *Obstetrics & Gynecology* in 2006 found it was equally as effective as hormone replacement therapy for some menopause symptoms, including hot flashes. And it did so without any serious side effects. Other studies, however, have found less promising results – and some have found no results at all.

So what's behind the conflicting findings? Well one idea speaks to the fact that for some women, other lifestyle factors capable of affecting hot flashes are diminishing the results. These include caffeine, tobacco, and alcohol, to name just a few.

And in this respect, my Hot Flash Solutions Lifestyle Diary could prove to be an enormous help in tracking down whatever factors may be conflicting with your personal success in using not only black cohosh, but any of the other natural solutions presented here.

But equally important is to recognize is that *not all black cohosh is created equal*. Indeed, many believe the success of this treatment is intimately tied to the specific black cohosh formulation you chose. The reason: Like all medications, how well it works is dependent on the level of active compounds it contains – in this case, the amount of triterpenoid glycosides.

To date, the vast majority of the clinical trials reporting menopause symptom relief using black cohosh were conducted using a single brand name supplement known as Remifemin.

In fact, Remifemin has been the subject of over 90 scientific papers, with some 20 clinical trials on over 3,000 women – and nearly all reported favorable results. In my research this is also the brand most often recommend by doctors.

Brand new to the Remifemin family is the "Good Night" version – designed to not only reduce hot flashes and night sweats, but also help you sleep better and more deeply.

In addition to black cohosh it also contains several of the most powerful herbal sleep aids around, including valerian, lemon balm and hops.

Studies show this particular blend can improve "night time" menopause issues, by some 88%, including trouble falling asleep, staying asleep, and reduced sleep quality. It is non-habit forming and helps gently support the body's natural sleep rhythms. Full benefits occur within 4 to 12 weeks.

Although once difficult to locate in the United States, today Remifemin products are relatively easy to find, frequently available in most health food stores and even some pharmacies.

But if you do have a problem finding it in your area, or you simply want to try an alternative brand, to combat hot flashes effectively make certain you chose a product that is labeled "standardized" and contains at least  20mg of root extract with 1mg of triterpene glycoside 27- deoxyactin (or 26-deoxyactin) per tablet.  This is the key formulation used in Remifemin and the one that clinical studies have been shown to work.

The average dose of black cohosh most effective for menopause-related symptoms ranges between 40mg and 80 mg daily, but you'll likely need to experiment within that framework to find the dose right for you.

How quickly should you see results? According to published reports, you should begin to see a difference in your hot flashes and some other menopause symptoms, within 4 to 12 weeks.

That said, remember that every woman is different – and every menopause is unique. So if you don't fall within that time frame, talk to your doctor about changing the dosing.

## BLACK COHOSH: 3 IMPORTANT CAUTIONS

### 1. LIVER TOXICITY

It's important to note that some preliminary research has linked black cohosh to liver toxicity, particularly in women with a past history of liver disease, including hepatitis C. At greatest risk are those who may have a silent, undiagnosed form of this disease. To date there have been approximately 30 cases of suspected liver toxicity problems linked to black cohosh, and one death. While many believe the evidence is still largely unsubstantiated, until we know more it's wise to discuss your intent to use black cohosh with your doctor, and if necessary, have a blood screening for liver malfunction both before you start treatment and perhaps midway through your regimen.

### 2. TERM OF USE

The safety studies conducted on black cohosh have never lasted longer than 6 months – so it's important that initially you confine your use to that time frame. That said, many doctors have suggested that it's okay to stop for a few months and then resume treatment again for another six months. Since there is no credible research on the estrogen impact of this herb beyond six months of continuous use, if you have a history of breast or endometrial (uterine) cancer, or if you are at high risk for either disease always check with your doctor before starting your initial 6 months of treatment, and again if you plan to use it for a second six month period.

### 3. DRUG INTERACTIONS

You should not use black cohosh if you are taking any SERM drugs – selective estrogen receptor modulators – including Tamoxifen used in the treatment of breast cancer, or raloxifene commonly used to improve bone health. There is some evidence to show that black cohosh competes with these medications for the same estrogen receptor - and if the herb gets there first, the benefits of the drug may be reduced.

## RED CLOVER:
## THE AGE-OLD BRAND NEW TREATMENT

When it comes to the treatment of hot flashes, among the most popular today is that which stems from the red clover plant. A cousin to the soybean, red clover is also a legume, containing some compounds similar to what is found in chick peas and lentils.

My grandmother, who was a midwife in rural Pennsylvania in the 1930's and 40's often spoke of the powerful properties of red clover on the female reproductive system, and frequently used it to help women overcome a variety of hormone-related problems.

Today, Grandma Ann's knowledge has come full circle with many medical studies now validating not only the fact that red clover is a potent treatment for many hormone-related conditions – including hot flashes – but also explaining why it works so well.

The reason: Isoflavones. Yes, the very same natural compound that makes soy so helpful for women during menopause is also found in the Red Clover plant – but in much greater abundance.

Indeed, the leaves of the Red Clover plant are brimming with not just two isoflavones as found in soy – genistein and daidzein - but also two others known as biochanin A and formononetin. And it is these two additional isoflavones that many believe give red clover its outstanding estrogenic effects.

In addition, red clover also works as an "adaptogen". So, when estrogen levels are low, red clover works like estrogen's "understudy" - taking on not only its characteristics, but also some of its duties in our body. This includes attaching to estrogen receptors in a way that "tricks" the body into believing all is right in hormone-land! The end result: Fewer symptoms such as hot flashes and night sweats.

But if you remember, earlier in this book you learned that it's not just low estrogen levels that can cause menopause symptoms. It's actually the *waxing and waning* of our hormones that creates the most troubling symptoms. And this is where red clover can really shine.

Why? It's the ability of this herb to adapt to what your body needs. So, when estrogen levels are too high, red clover becomes what doctors call a "down regulating" treatment. This means that by landing on and taking up a good portion of the estrogen receptors in your body, it keeps you from receiving too much of your own estrogen stimulation the way you might if those receptor sites were not blocked. In this way red clover may help keep your body from an estrogen overload. This is important for two reasons. First, it results in better hormone balance, which in the end is also what helps to alleviate many menopause symptoms, but particularly hot flashes and night sweats.

But even more importantly, it also means red clover may have some anti-cancer effects. By keeping receptors in the tissue of the breast and uterus from being over-stimulated by the presence of too much estrogen, it may help prevent or at least reduce the risk of breast and uterine cancer.

## RED CLOVER: THE BEST SOURCES

Although red clover is a legume, you don't eat it the way would a soybean. That said, if you've spent any time at all in health food store, then you know there is no shortage of ways to ingest this plant. From teas, to infusions, to various dried red clover leaf products, there appears to be a wide variety of choice.

Unfortunately, choosing a red clover product is not quite as easy as it looks. A variety of factors including varying levels of the key isoflavone constituents, as well as the conditions under which the plants are grown, when in their life cycle they are harvested, and the portion of the plant that is used in the red clover preparation (the leaves vs. the flowers vs. a combination of both) can impact effectiveness to an important degree. For this reason many believe the most reliable and the most effective form of red clover comes not as a food but as a supplement. And among those available, the one on which most studies have been done is "Promensil".

Each tablet of Promensil is standardized to contain a total of 40 mg of the four key isoflavones, (*genistein, daidzein, formononetin and biochanin A*), plus another form of weak plant estrogen called *coumestrol - and* all come directly from the red clover plant, with no chemical synthesization.

Thus far, research on more than 1,000 women worldwide shows it's a formulation that appears to work. In at least four of those studies – conducted by Tufts University School of Medicine, NYU School of Medicine, and Oxford University in England – women using Promensil experienced a significant reduction in hot flashes and night sweats.

In another study published in the European menopause journal *Maturitas* in 2002 researchers from the Netherlands found that taking 80mg of Promensil daily significantly reduced menopausal hot flashes when compared with placebo during a 1 year clinical trial. By the end of the 12 months, the women taking the red clover compound saw a 44 percent reduction in their hot flashes compared to almost no reduction in the placebo group.

More recently a study also published in Maturitas in 2006 reviewed 17 published clinical trials on red clover and concluded that not only was it effective in combating hot flashes, the more hot flashes a woman had, the better the product worked. Perhaps even more important is research showing that while Promensil acts like an estrogen in terms of mediating menopausal symptoms, it does so without increasing breast tissue density or the thickness of the uterine lining - both of which can occur with traditional estrogen therapy. And that means Promensil is not likely to increase the risk of cancer in these areas.

Other studies have suggested red clover may also have a positive effect on cholesterol, bone density and memory –acting much like estrogen to protect a woman's bones and heart, but again, without any of the side effects.

### RED CLOVER: HOW MUCH DO YOU NEED

If you are using Promensil as your main source of isoflavone, experts suggest one 40 mg capsule daily for mild to moderate symptoms, with up to 2 capsules daily for severe symptoms.

There is also an extra strength 80 mg capsule for easy once a day dosing.

If hot flashes are worse during the day, take Promensil with breakfast; if night sweats and night flashes are a bigger problem, take it at bedtime. You should see results in 2 to 5 weeks.

The newest red clover product, called Promensil Vitality combines 40mg of isoflavone with 500 mg of calcium and 3.5 mcg of vitamin D for extra bone health.

## RED CLOVER: WHAT YOU SHOULD KNOW

While studies have shown there to be no significant adverse effects from using Promensil or other forms of red clover, it's important to point out there are few studies longer than one year. So, use beyond that time, and particularly when taken in conjunction with a high-soy diet, has not been evaluated – either for effectiveness or safety.

Moreover, in certain situations there are some precautions about red clover you should heed. According to experts from the University of Maryland Medical Center pay attention to the following:

**Interactions and Depletions -** Red clover can interfere with the body's ability to process certain medications that require liver enzymes for proper breakdown. If you are taking any prescription medications or over-the-counter drugs on a regular basis, (particularly pain killers, tranquillizers, anti-depressants, or sleeping aids), talk to your doctor before taking any red clover supplements.

**Estrogens, hormone replacement therapy, birth control pills -** Because Promensil or any form of red clover exhibit estrogen-like effects it stands to reason that it may alter the effects of any drugs or supplements which contain or act on hormones. Again, check with your doctor before taking this supplement.

**Tamoxifen:** Red clover does appear to interfere with the activity of the anti-cancer drug Tamoxifen.

**Blood Thinners:** Red clover can enhance the effect of drugs used to thin the blood, as well as impacting herbs and supplements with blood-thinning properties, such as ginkgo, ginger, garlic and vitamin E. Don't mix them without your doctor's okay.

**Diabetes Drugs:** Because red clover can lower blood sugar, it can alter the effects of drugs used to control diabetes. If you are taking insulin or any other related drug for blood sugar, or if you are controlling your diabetes via diet, be certain to check with your doctor before taking Promensil or any red clover product.

Moreover, the makers of Promensil (Novagen) also warn that antibiotics may disrupt the "good bacteria" in the tummy necessary to properly absorb Promensil.

To prevent a reduced effect, add yogurt to your diet - which is actually a very good idea whenever you are taking antibiotics, since they  have been known to destroy the "good " bacteria necessary to gut health.

Additionally, you may see a reduced effect from Promensil if you are taking drugs for acid reflux, such as Zantac and Tazac, as well as medications such as Somac, Zoton, and Nexium.

## REPLACING HRT WITH PROMENSIL

Are you currently taking HRT - but looking to cut down or eliminate it? While your body will need a period of adjustment before you can begin gaining the benefits of Promensil, according to research conducted by the company, here's what you can try:

- Take both HRT and Promensil (one tablet daily) together for a period of time, before gradually reducing the dose of HRT.
- Stop HRT and start Promensil twice daily (or until menopause symptoms are managed), then 1 tablet thereafter.
- Stop HRT and start Promensil one tablet daily. However, there may be significant menopause symptoms associated with an abrupt changeover until your body adjusts.

## DONG QUAI:
## THE CONTROVERSIAL HOT FLASH HERB

If you look to the history of traditional Chinese medicine (TCM) perhaps no herb has a more impressive record of successfully treating hot flashes than Dong Quai, in use in China for over 2,000 years.

Fast-forward to modern times, and studies published in both 1963 and again in 1984 further detailed its success as a menopause treatment. The key compound found in Dong Quai- "ferulic acid"- was shown to have an impact on hot flashes, decreasing both intensity and frequency. Unfortunately more modern research has challenged those findings.

A study published in 1997 in the journal *Fertility and Sterility* found the recommended dosage of Dong Quai – 4.5 mg daily – had no greater effect on hot flashes or vaginal tissue shrinkage than a sugar pill placebo. Moreover one database search conducted by Columbia University found no convincing clinical evidence of any kind that Dong Quai was effective in treating any menopause symptoms.

But Chinese medicine doctors – who continue to prescribe Dong Quai for hot flashes – say the reason behind the conflicting results is that this herb should *never be used on its own*, but instead combined with at least 4 other herbs for what is known as a "synergistic effect".

Essentially, they believe the "whole" is greater than the sum of its parts and together these herbs accomplish something that cannot be achieved when they are used singularly.

Moreover, traditional Chinese medicine formulations typically contain much higher doses of Dong Quai than what are found in western treatment regimens.

The bottom line: If you want to give Dong Quai a try, look to a traditional Chinese medicine specialist for a product recommendation – or at the very least seek out a combination product specifically designed for hot flashes, one that contains Dong Quai in conjunction with other herbs.

**IMPORTANT CAUTION:** Dong Quai increases photosensitivity, so you may experience a rash if you go out in bright sunlight while taking this herb. Dong Quai should also be avoided if you are taking the blood thinning medication Warfarin.

## CHASTEBERRY –WHAT YOU SHOULD KNOW

Also known as "vitex", the herb Chasteberry is believed to impact hot flashes by regulating some hormones that impact both the hypothalamus and pituitary glands. Working through these brain centers it is believed to also impact the production of progesterone, which, as you read earlier , may also play a role in hot flashes.

In two surveys of some 1,500 German women, 40 drops of Vitex daily for 166 days relieved symptoms related to progesterone deficiency – but the kind more often seen in women who experience PMS rather than menopause. This included relief from fluid retention, bloating, breast tenderness, headache, and fatigue, with relief occurring in about 3 weeks.

While some researchers continue to believe chasteberry can also help decrease hot flashes, depression and vaginal dryness, currently the German E Commission recommends Chasteberry only for menstrual disorders and painful breasts. The suggested dosage is 20mg daily.

**Caution:** Pharmacist Suzy Cohen, R.Ph, says that if you have suffered from endometriosis, (a menstrual related disorder), fibroid tumors, or cancer of the breast, ovaries or uterus, don't use Chasteberry until

you check with your doctor. The hormone activity associated with this herb could worsen your symptoms and possibly interfere with treatments or prevention strategies.

## VITAMIN E & CITRUS BIOFLAVONOID

Although they are not considered herbs, both vitamin E and bioflavonoids are certainly natural and many women report they have among the best flash-controlling properties of anything Mother Nature can offer. In addition, there is some evidence to show they can help with vaginal dryness as well as reduce mood swings and anxiety associated with perimenopause and menopause changes. Essentially, bioflavonoids are natural compounds found in fruits and vegetables and, along with Vitamin C (another hot flash nutrient), they are extremely plentiful in citrus fruits like oranges, lemons and grapefruit.

The veggies containing the highest level of bioflavonoids include carrots, squash, tomatoes, berries, broccoli, and other greens.

Since most of us don't eat enough fruits to get an adequate amount of these nutrients, pharmacist Suzy Cohen, R.Ph suggests supplements containing 500 to 1,000 IUs of mixed vitamin E daily (that's a supplement that contains many forms of vitamin E) along with 1,000 mg of bioflavonoids daily.

Cohen says the most important bioflavonoid is called "HMC hesperiden" so check your supplement label to make sure it's included.

## THE HERBS THAT DON'T WORK

Although there are many herbal products that claim to control hot flashes, most are not backed up by medical research. Here is a short list of the some of the more popular recommended herbs that don't appear to live up to their reputation.

GINSENG – Experience with ginseng is typified by the results of one Norwegian study of 400 women who took this herb, or a placebo, for 16 weeks. While the women reported feeling better overall, with less depression, unfortunately their hot flashes weren't affected.

WILD YAM SUPPLEMENTS - A cousin to the sweet potato this supplement has enjoyed a long history as a natural source of compounds that the body converts into progesterone. Unfortunately that conversion process cannot actually take place in the body. A study published in the medical journal *Climacteric* in 2001 reported that wild yam supplements had no greater impact on menopause symptoms than a placebo.

EVENING OIL OF PRIMROSE – An important source of omega 3 and omega 6 fatty acids and a powerful natural anti-inflammatory compound, Evening Oil of Primrose is often suggested as a treatment for a variety of reproductive problems with some success. However, as a treatment for hot flashes, you're bound to be disappointed. One six month study published in the *British Medical Journal* in 1994 women reported a slight decrease in night sweats after using this supplement, there was no effect on hot flashes.

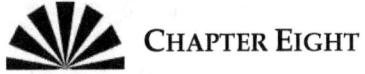 CHAPTER EIGHT

# Aromatherapy For Hot Flashes

If you've ever smelled a lovely flower or a favorite perfume and found that it uplifted your mood, or even made you feel more relaxed, then you have already experienced a form of aromatherapy.

Clinically speaking, aromatherapy is the "science" of using fragrance to stimulate or calm certain areas of the brain, most often those that play a role in stress, anxiety, and mood.

But the more commonly known type of aromatherapy involves using scented oils and plant based natural fragrances help enhance feelings of well-being and reduce stress. Indeed, there are now numerous studies published in top medical journals showing that aromatherapy is an effective way to reduce stress – which, as you will read in just few minutes, does play a role in hot flashes.

But more importantly there is a growing body of medical evidence to show that certain aromatherapy formulations may have a direct impact on menopausal symptoms – including hot flashes.

In one study published very recently in the journal *Evidence-based Complimentary and Alternative Medicine* a group of Korean researchers found that an aromatherapy massage using essences of lavender, geranium, rose and jasmine in almond and primrose oils once a week for 8 weeks, significantly reduced a variety of menopausal symptoms, including hot flashes.

What is less clear, however, is whether the women benefited from the fragrant oils, the massage, or the combination!

In a second study published in the *Journal of Alternative Medicine* a group of Japanese researchers found that two consultations with an aroma therapist, followed by one month of at-home aromatherapy was also effective in reducing menopause symptoms, including hot flashes.

So evidence is starting to mount that aromatherapy may be helpful for some women, at least on a short term or immediate basis.

## CLARY SAGE- THE HOT FLASH SCENT

Among the most popular aromatherapy essences specifically for hot flashes is Clary Sage. A flowering plant native to France, Italy and Syria but now grown worldwide it features unique heart shaped leaves and pale blue, purple, or pink flowers that fully blossom from May through September. It is the blossoms and the leaves that are steam distilled down to clear or light yellow colored oil. The aroma is slightly sweet, with a fresh, clean scent, which some say has nutty balsamic undertones.

Clary Sage essential oil can be mixed with any carrier oil – like almond or primrose – and then used for massage, or simply to smell when you feel a hot flash coming on. The oil of Clary Sage can also be distilled down further into scented "water" which can be used much like a fragrant room or body spray.

Another popular aromatherapy facial spray is rosewater. Available in many cosmetic and health food stores, there are no studies to show it works, but anecdotally many women report it helps reduce tension, cools skin, and reduces the severity of hot flashes.

Other essential oils thought to be beneficial for reducing stress and helping menopause symptoms include:

- Bergamot – to lift spirits, reduce anxiety and alleviate depression.

- Chamomile, to ease anxiety and tension headaches.

- Geranium, to help rebalance hormones and reduce stress.

- Jasmine for tension and anxiety.

- Juniper to relieve water retention.

- Lavender –for relaxation and promote deep, healthy sleep.

### ONE WORD OF CAUTION ...

Essential oils are complex and strong compounds and should never be applied directly to the skin. Always dilute essential oils with"carrier" oils, like almond, jojoba or primrose.

In addition you can also purchase essential oils that are already distilled down to fragrant waters. The scent isn't quite as strong as an essential oil, but they can be easier to use and definitely easier to travel with. You can keep a small spray bottle in your purse and spray whenever you feel the need for some "flash relief".

As a bonus, many women find that a rosewater spray not only cools a flash, but also hydrates the skin, increases moisture content, and increases the effectiveness of moisturizers. So, you not only feel better, you smell great – and you look great! What's not to love?

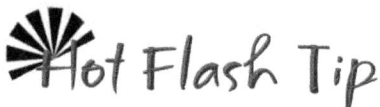

For quick hot flash relief when you're on the go carry a migraine cool patch!

These ultra thin portable gel packs provide instant cool with no refrigeration needed.

Just unwrap it and place it on the back of your neck , or on the inside of your elbow or wrist to instantly cool you down and  reset your thermostat. Brands include Wellpatch and Kool Patch .

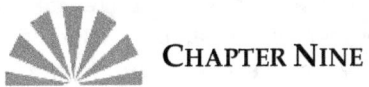

**CHAPTER NINE**

# The Stress Solution: What You Must Know!

If you're like most women who experience hot flashes, you know they have a way of occurring at the most inopportune moments: Just as you arrive at that fabulous cocktail party, when you're about to give an important business presentation, when you're meeting your daughter's future in-laws for the first time. In fact, whenever you're under pressure to look, feel or be your best, out of the blue that burning red hot flash arrives.

But the very fact that your flashes frequently occur when you are in a stressful situation should give you a very good clue about one important link.

And if you guessed stress, you're right!

Indeed, stress can affect your menopause body in myriad ways – from making you feel jittery, tired, achy, and frightened to feeling hot and sweaty - *and not in a good way!*

In fact, one of the primary body systems linked to stress is the autonomic nervous system – which, when it gets the cue we are excited, can begin pouring out hormones that not only make us perspire but can also impact body temperature.

During the midlife years stress can double these effects. Indeed, many of the same hormones involved in the stress response – like cortisol and norepinephrine – can also impact hormones like estrogen, and vice versa.

When stress becomes chronic the effects on your body can increase, so much so that menopausal symptoms can worsen. In fact, Harvard University professor and stress expert Dr. Alice Domar believes that the effects of stress on our hormone activity can be so great, it can even incite hot flashes – or certainly cause them to occur more frequently and with more intensity.

In one 6 year study of some 400 menopausal women doctors from the University of Pennsylvania found that those who had the highest levels of anxiety (as measured in blood tests of stress hormones) experienced 5 *times the number of hot flashes* as women who were *less anxious*. The study was published in the journal *Menopause*.

Many experts believe that one link is the system that produces adrenal hormones. Indeed when your life is hectic, when you literally "bite off more than you can chew" you are continually asking your adrenal glands to pour out the hormones that give you the energy to go-go-GO!

But just like a bank account, where constant withdrawals and no deposits can cause your funds to run dry, so too can your adrenal glands "run dry". Indeed, when you continue to stress them non-stop, eventually they will burn out. When they do you won't only feel exhausted all the time, you'll also get more hot flashes.

Indeed, one little known fact is that adrenal glands have a direct link to your body's internal thermostat. Burn out your adrenal glands and your internal thermostat is no longer as effective in telling your body when to cool down. The end result: The more you push yourself, the more stress you experience, and the worse your hot flashes can be.

## HOW STRESSED ARE YOU? A QUICK TEST!

While most of us can sense when our stress levels are getting out of control, what is harder to detect is just how close we are to actual adrenal burnout – or if we have already crossed the line.

One thing you can look out for is fatigue – a sense of tiredness that doesn't seem to go away even when you think you're getting enough sleep.

But according to registered pharmacist Suzy Cohen, R.PH, author of "The 24 Hour Pharmacist" even using fatigue as a guide, many women still overlook adrenal exhaustion as a potential problem. To make sure you know everything you need to know about your mid-life body, Cohen recommends the following easy "Stress Test" you can take at home.

**THE STRESS TEST**

Sit in front of a mirror in a darkened room and shine a flashlight into your eyes for about a minute.

When you're done you can turn on the lights and look in the mirror- specifically at your eyes.

If the pupils are tiny – smaller than normal – and they stay that way for at least a little while, then you have not yet reached the point of adrenal exhaustion.

If, on the other hand, your pupil size rapidly changes back and forth from tiny to dilated several times, then you are likely suffering at least some significant level of adrenal fatigue – and a sure sign you've got to do something immediately to reduce your stress.

## REDUCE STRESS & SAY "BAH BYE " HOT FLASHES!

No matter how stressed you might be, the good news is that taking steps to reduce the tension and anxiety in your life can also help restore your adrenal gland function to normal, and in the process reduce your hot flashes!

Okay…so I know this is a lot easier said than done - particularly when the situations that are causing the most stress are those that are out of your control.

But even if you can't change the situations – a miserable boss, a teenage son-gone-suddenly-wild, aging parents that are increasingly difficult to care for - you *can still take steps to help your body handle the stress you are experiencing,* and in that way reduce its effects.

> •In one recent study, published in *Menopause: The Journal of the North American Menopause Society,* researchers found that those women who participated in an 11 week stress reducing program reduced their incidence of hot flashes overall by some 39%. And even in the women who continued to have some hot flashes severity was decreased by 40%!

As an extra bonus – 28% of the women also reported an improvement in the overall quality of their life – and an improved ability to cope with all their menopause symptoms.

## MEDITATE …& GET FEWER HOT FLASHES!

While it's easy to recognize stress in our lives, it's not always so easy to reduce it. This is particularly true if you believe the only way to control stress is to control stressful situations in your life.

But if you haven't already figured this part out, this is probably the least effective way to relieve your stress. In fact, studies show that trying to control stressful situations often increases our anxiety – which in turn can lead to even more hot flashes.

What's a lot easier is learning to control *your reaction to stress*. When you do that, you naturally reduce its effects on your body – which has very much the same end result as getting rid of the stress itself. Moreover, once you learn to control how your body reacts to stress, you'll not only reduce your hot flashes, you'll improve your overall health, reducing your risk of heart disease, high blood pressure, even some cancers.

Among the best places to start: Meditation, yoga, and deep breathing. All three work in similar ways to help calm your autonomic nervous system, and reduce the production of stress hormones and chemicals that can feed your anxiety and, over time, reduce your hot flashes.

Indeed, in one study published in the journal *Menopause* researchers found that meditation dramatically reduced hot flashes in women who were "on fire" on average, 7 times a day.

## The Meditations That Work

The following were the types of meditations used in the study:

***Progressive Body Scan Meditation:*** To try this, lie on your back in a relaxed, comfortable position (either on the floor, in bed, in a chaise lounge, etc.) and gradually concentrate on each area of your body, from head to toe.

Think about how each body part feels, and what kind of sensations you feel at each major point along the way. Don't try to diagnose any pains or reason behind any sensations – just experience them as you move from one area to the next.

*SITTING MEDITATIONS:* This involves sitting in a comfortable position – either on the floor, on pillows, in bed, on a couch or a chair – and focusing on your breathing and bodily sensations. Don't try to control how your body feels, just let it be, concentrating on how your blood flows effortlessly through your body, how your breathing continues, how your muscles relax.

*MINDFUL STRETCHING* - This is a more active form of meditation that many women who can't sit still find easy to do. In this instance comfortably stretch various parts of your body – your arms, legs, neck, shoulders and torso - and with each stretch concentrate on the sensations you are feeling in each area of your body, blocking out all other thoughts.

## TAKE A BREATH …
## KISS YOUR HOT FLASH GOODBYE!

Another popular form of mediation involves deep breathing – a way of controlling the length and depth of each breath you take for a controlled period of time. How can this help? First, when you breathe shallow – gasping small bits of air quickly and frequently - you can throw your body into hyperventilation mode. This is a condition where you actually take in too much oxygen. This can not only make you feel dizzy and lightheaded, but also bring on a hot flash – or exacerbate one you're already having.

Conversely, learning to take deeper, longer breaths can not only reduce hyperventilation, it can also give you an automatic stress reduction skill you can use anytime, anywhere, to cut anxiety and tension. But perhaps most important is research showing that deep breathing exercises can significantly reduce the incidence of hot flashes almost as effectively as certain types of hormone therapy!

In one study published in the *Journal of Psychosomatic Obstetrics and Gynecology* doctors found that just 10 to 20 minutes of "paced breathing" per day for several weeks dramatically decreased the intensity of hot flashes as well as decreasing anxiety, depression, and overall body tension.

In another medical study, an overview published in the *American Journal of Medicine,* researchers documented results from 3 controlled studies showing that deep breathing – or "paced respiration" – reduced hot flashes by nearly 50% with no adverse effects! Some hormone therapy only offers a 40% reduction!

## YOUR DEEP BREATHING PRIMER

According to a number of studies, the method of deep breathing that appeared to be most effective in reducing hot flashes is known as "paced respiration".

Here's how to give it a try:

1. Find a cool, quiet environment, with a comfortable chair. You can also sit on the floor or in bed – whatever feels relaxing.

2. Set a timer for a specific period – say 15 minutes.

3. Once you are comfortably seated, close your eyes.

4. Concentrate on relaxing all your muscles. Begin with your feet and work your way up your body, concentrating on how each muscle group feels when it's loose and relaxed.

5. Once you feel your body start to loosen up, start focusing on your breathing. Breathe naturally – through your nose - at the same rate your normally breathe, but simply concentrate on each inhale and exhale.

6. When you are comfortable with this, inhale, then exhale, and then quietly says the word "one" to yourself.

7. Keep repeating this until your timer goes off.

If at first you don't feel relaxed, or you tense your body while you're breathing, don't worry. The longer you practice, the more relaxed you will become. You can also expect idle thoughts to enter your mind while you're breathing – including stressful thoughts, work or financial worries, home or family concerns.

Just keep concentrating on your breathing and try to replace those thoughts with visuals of each inhale and exhale. For example, visualize a green meadow with each inhale, a blue sky with each exhale – whatever scene, color and atmosphere you find relaxing.

When you are done, open your eyes, and sit quietly for a few moments before standing up.

*Tip: To make deep breathing exercises easier – or to help control hot flashes while you are exercising – try a Breathe Right Nasal Strip. They hold open nasal passages and I've found they encourage deeper, more restful breathing.*

## THE YOGA SOLUTION

It's been embraced by movie stars, touted as the saving grace by super models and enjoyed by tens of thousands of regular folks for decades. It's yoga – and it's not only taking credit for helping to tone and shape the body, but also reduce stress and even improve our outlook on life.

More recently however, yoga is quietly garnering a whole new slew of fans – women suffering from hot flashes and night sweats. And many are reporting they are finding relief! Indeed, research that is ongoing – and some already completed – continues to show that women who practice yoga have fewer hot flashes, and the ones they do have are likely to pass more quickly and be less intense, when compared to women who do a different form of exercise.

Yoga also seems able to impact night sweats, improve sleep quality and even improve memory in women going through menopause.

•In one study published in the journal *Maturitas* researchers from the University of Washington found that women who took one 60 minute hatha yoga class per week, for 7 to 10 weeks, and practiced at home for about fifteen minutes a day significantly reduced their incidence of not only hot flashes, they reported sleeping better as well – with fewer night sweats and awakenings.

- In another report recently issued by a group of Indian researchers, women who practiced yoga for 8 weeks saw a significant reduction in a variety of menopause-related symptoms including not only hot flashes, but also night sweats and other sleep disturbances.

Interestingly the study also found that yoga seemed to help with memory problems as well, another temporary but irritating symptom of menopause.

As convincing as the research is, however, some women still shy away from yoga, believing it requires putting your body in contorted positions or even going into a "trance" in order to gain benefits.

If you're one of these yoga-shy gals, fear not! Most of the yoga exercises that yield the best hot flash results require only simple body postures and very little stress and strain!

As for the trance aspect...not to worry! You won't be leaving the earth any time soon! The goal of yoga is to relax your mind and your body – but trust me, if your cell phone rings you'll hear it!

If you do decide to give yoga a try, I would advise that you either join a class or at the very least purchase an instructional DVD. I like the video explanations better than the books since they offer you a good visual that can make yoga workouts easier to understand.

You can find suggestions for inexpensive yoga videos at www.YourMenopause.com. Or check your local library – many now have a nice selection.

To help get you started right now, what follows is a quick primer on the different types of yoga and a little bit about what they involve. It's a good idea to familiarize yourself with the different types – so you know what kinds of videos or books to look for.

## YOUR YOGA PRIMER

Although in America – and even parts of Europe – yoga is considered a type of exercise, its roots actually encompass an entire lifestyle philosophy that was practiced by devout members of the Hindu faith beginning about 5,000 years ago. Their regimen included not only yoga postures and meditation but also a strict diet, and performing random acts of kindness.

Today, however, yoga is viewed primarily as a form of physical exercise and a way to relax. Often it is combined with meditation and deep breathing exercises to achieve what yoga enthusiasts call a balanced harmony between body, mind, and spirit. If that sounds a little too "new age-y" for you, relax! It's really all about reducing stress on both a mental and a physical level.

There are numerous types of yoga being practiced, each with its own postures and philosophies. What follows are the four most popular forms of this exercise.

## HATHA Yoga

Known as the "traditional " form of yoga, it is by far the most popular type practiced in the US – and it's known for its gentle simple movements. However, because "hatha yoga" is really the generic term used to describe the movement and posture segment of the yoga lifestyle, the actual movements used can vary from class to class depending on who is doing the teaching. Still, finding a hatha yoga class is a good place to begin your yoga journey!

## IYENGAR Yoga

Although more rigorous than the more common type of hatha yoga, it shares some of the same techniques particularly in regard to body alignment and postures. Depending on who is teaching the class the movements can still be gentle, focusing mostly on flexibility and the meditative aspects of yoga. Iyengar yoga has been used in a number of menopause symptom studies with good results. If you find a class offering iyengar yoga, and you've never tried this form of exercise before, make sure it's a class for beginners.

## BIKRAM Yoga

This is clearly a more advanced form of yoga that involves practicing various postures in high heat temperatures – like rooms heated to as much as 100 degrees. Obviously, not a great choice if you're looking to reduce hot flashes! The purpose of the high heat is to aid in muscle stretching and allow the use of more complex postures. All totaled it involves a routine of 26 different poses that can be difficult for beginners to achieve. I'd stay away from this one !

**ASHTANGA Yoga**

This is not for the faint of heart - or the weak of muscle! Also known as "power yoga" it is the most physically demanding of all the yoga types and requires fast paced movement and strong breathing skills. Again, not good choices as a way of dealing with hot flashes – and definitely not a good choice if you are a "yoga virgin". Still, it can be something to work towards – and it is a great body conditioning, that's for sure!

## Aerobics, Stress & Hot Flashes: What Can Help

For most of us it seems like the absolute worst thing you can do to cool down is aerobic exercise! I mean after all, if your face and neck aren't on fire before you start, certainly all that jumping and jiving is sure to kick off those body temperature snafus and throw you into an instant heat.

But as intuitive as *that sounds*, it seems studies have shown the opposite! Regular aerobic exercise – that which increases your heart rate - not only reduces the level of stress hormones that play a role in hot flashes, it can also have a *stabilizing* effect on your body thermostat.

More specifically, it can help calm down the vaso-motor system that sets a hot flash in motion – so fewer hot flashes are likely to occur.

In fact, exercise has been found to be so effective as a way to combat hot flashes, it is recommended by the North American Menopause Society as an effective tool. And studies seem to show it really works!

- In one Scandinavian study published in their journal of obstetrics and gynecology, researchers found that women who exercise regularly not only have fewer hot flashes overall, but those that do occur are less severe and end more quickly than those experienced by women who don't work out.

- In another study researchers found that blood levels of estrogen actually increase directly following 20 to 30 minutes of aerobic exercise – and they remain elevated for a number of hours afterwards. In this study, published in the journal *Medical Science in Sports Exercise* 55% of the women who exercised regularly found relief from hot flashes. As you learned earlier, the more stable your estrogen levels, the less likely it is for your hypothalamus gland to trigger a hot flash.

- In still another study published in the *New England Journal of Medicine,* not only was exercise proven to reduce hot flashes but when the women also began taking calcium supplements daily, their flashes decreased even further!

If you are battling depression *and* menopause symptoms at the same time, the news is even better. Exercise can help both problems simultaneously.

In a Harvard study of moods and cycles published in the journal *Menopause,* research on some 500 women revealed those who were suffering from clinical depression found exercise reduced hot flashes and other vasomotor symptoms, when compared to sedentary women who did no exercise. Not to mention the fact that the exercise also had a positive effect on their depression symptoms.

Moreover, research also shows that regular workouts can reduce related menopause symptoms including mood swings and sleepless nights – which have also been known to increase the severity of hot flashes during your waking hours.

## THE WORKOUT TO REDUCE HOT FLASHES

Certainly not every exercise regimen is right for every woman. Indeed, by midlife many of us are dealing with arthritis, and various kinds of aches and pains including some, like knee pain, resulting from too many workouts when we were younger. But that said, Dr. Mona Shangold, Director for Women's Health and Sports Gynecology in Philadelphia, Pennsylvania, advises that if it's possible, the best midlife exercise prescription includes:

•**Aerobics:** 20 minutes, 3 days of week.
Try: brisk walking, riding a stationary or regular bike, swimming, rowing, dancing.

•**Resistance**: 20 minutes, 3 times a week. Activities include: lifting weights, using rubber resistance bands, using exercise machines that push against body force.

•**Stretching:** Every day! Just reach up and touch the sky, reach down and touch your toes, and generally stretch out the muscles in your body particularly before and after every workout.

**One Word Of Caution:**  While exercise may help reduce hot flashes in the long run, the circumstances under which you do your exercises – particularly the clothes you wear while exercising - could increase symptoms while you're working out.  Be sure to read the chapter on **Fashions and Flashes,** and the section on the links between your personal environment and hot flashes,  for more tips on how to exercise cool and comfortable.

## MORE WAYS TO REDUCE MENOPAUSE STRESS

In addition to the impact that physical activity can have on helping you handle stress, there are also a number of nutrients and herbs that have been shown to have a direct impact on the adrenal glands – and in that way, help combat stress and restore body, mind and spirit!  While you won't see the effects overnight, when used in conjunction with a stress-relieving exercise program, a healthy diet, and devoting more time to relaxation, over time you will see a difference. Not only are you likely to be more relaxed, you may also have fewer mood swings and anxiety attacks – and your hot flashes should be improving as well.

## THE HERBS FOR ADRENAL REPAIR

According to pharmacist Suzy Cohen, R.Ph, there are 5 herbs specifically associated with adrenal repair. Each is considered an "adaptogen" - meaning they regulate rather than speed up or slow down stress hormones. You can try them individually or combine them, but either way you'll need about 30 days before you will begin to see a measureable difference in how you feel.

### Herb:  Panax Ginseng
*Recommend Dosage:*  200mg, two to three times daily
**FYI:** If you develop acne or facial hair lower the dosage.


### Herb: Licorice Root
*Recommend Dosage:* 500-1,000 mg before meals and at bedtime 4 days per week.
**FYI**: Make sure your supplement contains "whole licorice"; the version known as "DGL" won't offer immune support. If you have high blood pressure, or any form of heart disease *do not use licorice root* unless you check with your doctor.


### Herb: Ashwagandha or "Indian ginseng"
*Recommend Dosage*: 400-500 mg  2 to 3  times daily.
**FYI:**    Reduces anxiety and increases sleep, and reduces arthritis pain and inflammation.


### Herb: Rhodiola Rose
*Recommended Dosage:* 50 – 100 mg twice daily.
**FYI:** This herb works to reduce anxiety, ease depression, and increase energy, by helping you to sleep better and more soundly.


### Herb: Cordyceps
*Recommend Dosage:* 300-400mg twice daily.
**FYI:** Frequently used by  endurance athletes and Olympic champions to help restore balance after intense workouts, this herb reduces  blood pressure, and help you to sleep better. Because it's from the "mushroom" family of plants, don't use it if you have a mushroom allergy.

## THE MENOPAUSE STRESS NUTRIENTS

In addition to eating a balanced diet with plenty of fresh fruits, vegetables and whole grains, there are also a handful of nutrients which many believe can have a positive, restorative effect on adrenal function - and in the process mediate stress and some symptoms of menopause. Here's what might help:

**Vitamin B 5:** Also known as pantothenic acid, this nutrient has a direct impact on adrenal function and fatigue. It can also help reduce the risk of infection and may have some impact on cholesterol. The best sources are grains, nuts, beans and yeast or daily supplements 500-1,000 mg.

**Vitamin C:** This is the ultimate stress vitamin! It not only helps the body to reduce stress hormones to normal after an isolated stressful event occurs, but because long term stress depletes vitamin C replenishing it with a supplement is important. This nutrient is also known as the "menopause vitamin" because when taken in conjunction with bioflavonoids (natural compounds that are plentiful in citrus fruits) studies show it reduces hot flashes.

In one study, supplements of 900 mg of hesperiden (a bioflavonoid) plus 1200 mg of vitamin C daily had a significant impact on hot flashes. If you have a sensitive tummy look for "buffered" vitamin C and take it in 500 mg doses.

**Vitamin E:** While the popularity of this vitamin has had its ups and downs, in terms of menopause the reports are generally good.

As early as the 1940's research has shown that it may reduce hot flashes, control mood swings and help with vaginal dryness. In terms of your adrenal glands, it won't have any specific effects but as part of your overall mid-life nutrient portrait it can help keep your body balanced – and that can help reduce the effects of stress.

**Vitamin D:** Although it plays no real role in adrenal gland function, because it's such an important vitamin for midlife it bears mentioning.

One reason is the link to bone health. As you read earlier, when we are young estrogen helps our bones absorb calcium – the mineral necessary to keep them strong. As estrogen levels drop, vitamin D can pick up the slack  - one reason it's essential to take during this time of life. Vitamin D also produces a protein called osteocalcin, which also plays a role in bone strength.

Estimates are that up to 80% of Americans are vitamin D deficient – and if you stay out of the sun you're probably one of them. To know for sure, ask your doctor for a blood test known as 25-OH.  This is the most reliable way of testing the amount of vitamin D circulating in your blood.

If you're low, supplement with up to 1,000 mg daily.

## ACUPUNCTURE & HOT FLASHES:  GOOD NEWS !

Acupuncture is an ancient Chinese medicine treatment that relies on the painless but strategic placement of tiny needles into a "grid-like" pattern that spans the body, from head to toe. The needles are used to stimulate certain key "energy points" believed to regulate spiritual, mental, emotional, and physical balance.

For most folks acupuncture is an effective way to relieve pain. But more recently research has shown it may also impact hot flashes. While doctors aren't exactly sure how or why, in the past it has it has been used to successfully treat a number of hormone-related problems, including infertility linked to ovulation problems.

As such, many now believe acupuncture reduces hot flashes by working on these same hormonal pathways, normalizing levels of reproductive hormones and balancing natural body chemicals involved in the reproductive cycle.

Another theory says acupuncture stimulates various neuro-chemical receptors in the brain linked to the central nervous system activity that controls a hot flash.

There is even some evidence that acupuncture may play a role in regulating the activity of the hypothalamus gland itself – which, as you read earlier, helps control, and regulate body temperature and mediate hot flashes. .

Regardless of how it works, research is beginning to mount that it clearly has beneficial effects on hot flashes, not only in women in the perimenopause and menopause years but also women with hot flashes related to hormonal breast cancer therapies.

In one very recent study conducted by doctors at the Henry Ford Hospital in Detroit, researchers found that acupuncture was just as effective as the antidepressant Effexor, in relieving hot flashes in breast cancer patients.

And while the women using acupuncture experienced no bad side effects, those taking Effexor reported bouts of nausea, headache, difficult sleeping, dizziness, increased blood pressure, fatigue and anxiety.

So it seems acupuncture may be more pleasant to endure as well as being more helpful. In fact, the women who received the acupuncture also reported an increase in energy, feelings of well being and sexual desire – as well as fewer hot flashes!

Perhaps the best news of all was that the relief not only lasted through the 12 weeks of acupuncture treatment, but a follow-up of 15 weeks showed the women were still experiencing the benefits!

Those taking the antidepressant stopped receiving benefits in just two weeks.

Indeed, doctors now estimate that having a few acupuncture treatments about 4 times a year might be all the average woman needs to feel good and control her hot flashes all year long.

This is particularly good news since many insurance plans now cover acupuncture treatments.

## ACUPUNCTURE HELPS NIGHT SWEATS

If its night sweats that represent your biggest menopause challenge, you'll be happy to know acupuncture can help here as well. In one study conducted at Stanford University and reported in the journal *Fertility and Sterility* doctors found acupuncture to be extremely effective in relieving night time hot flashes and night sweats by some 28% with just 7 treatments.

And here's a bonus: Studies recently published in the journal *Obstetrics & Gynecology* found acupuncture can also help control an over-active bladder, another common symptom of menopause. Indeed, in a randomized study women who received four weekly acupuncture treatments had significant improvements in bladder capacity, urgency, and frequency, and quality-of-life scores.

This led the authors to conclude that "In this study, acupuncture had a significant short-term effect on overactive bladder, similar in scope to the improvement offered by drug therapy and physical or behavioral therapy."

## CAN ACUPUNCTURE HELP YOU?

Statistically speaking, chances are you will find at least some relief from a round or two of acupuncture treatment. But that said, it's important to keep in mind that again, every woman is different, so the degree to which you find relief is largely personal.

But if in fact you do decide to give acupuncture a try, tantamount to finding hot flash relief is finding a qualified specialist to administer the treatment.

What should you look for? First, be certain to find a specialist that is adequately trained and licensed in acupuncture, as well as one who has a background in treating hot flashes resulting from menopause or those resulting from other causes, such as breast cancer treatments.

Indeed, an MD who simply practices acupuncture once in a while often has just several hundred hours of experience, compared to several thousand hours of training and practice required for a traditional Chinese doctor. Here are some other key things to focus on:

- Look for an acupuncturist associated with a major academic medical center.

- If you are undergoing cancer treatments make certain your oncologist has a working relationship with your acupuncturist, and that they work in harmony for your treatment regimen.

- If you are not seeing a gynecologist for the treatment of your menopause symptoms, it's a good idea to have at least one baseline checkup first – and let your doctor know you plan to seek acupuncture treatment.

Although acupuncture often works in harmony with Chinese herbal medicine, if you are using any prescribed hormone treatments, including natural hormones, or if you are taking any chemo-preventive drugs for breast cancer, do not take any Chinese herbs without the OK of your  oncologist or gynecologist.

If you experience any adverse symptoms while undergoing acupuncture, including an increase in uterine bleeding, a resumption of bleeding if your menstrual cycle has already stopped, or an increase in hot flashes or night sweats, stop treatment and speak with your gynecologist.

Finally, if you do decide to give acupuncture a try, make certain to run the idea by your doctor first.

Certainly, you might get some resistance – many western trained doctors are not as familiar with the practice as perhaps they should be – it's important that your doctor weigh in on any *medical* reasons why you should not participate in this therapy.

This is especially important if you have been diagnosed with breast, uterine or ovarian cancer, even if your treatment regimens are finished.  While it's likely that acupuncture will help you as well, still it's important for all your doctors to work in harmony, in order for you to benefit most from the expertise of each specialist.

# Hot Flash Tip

Choose your cheese wisely!
Aged cheeses like some Swiss, plus most cheddars,
provolone, Romano, parmesan, feta and edam
contain a natural chemical known as "tyramine"
which can impact the vasomotor system and in
some women bring on or exacerbate a hot flash.

Tyramine is also found in  fermented or marinated
foods including smoked fish, beef and poultry, as
well as  sour cream, shrimp paste, soy sauce,
teriyaki sauce, tofu, tempeh, miso  soup,
sauerkraut, fava beans, snow pea pods, avocados,
bananas, eggplant, figs, red plums, raspberries,
peanuts, Brazil nuts,  coconut,  most
processed sandwich meats, and yeast.

Tyramine is also found in red wine.
So, if you find that you get a hot flash after drinking
red wine but not white wine, beer or a whisky
cocktail, it's not the alcohol that's bothering you, it's
likely the tyramine. For many women, switching
from red to white wine dramatically decreases
hot flashes.

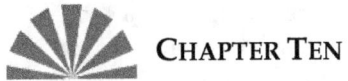 **Chapter Ten**

# The Natural Hormone Debate

Perhaps nothing has caused more of a stir in women's health then all of the recent attention placed on natural and bioidentical hormones – plant based compounds that some believe can offer the benefits of traditional hormone therapy without the risks.

If you're among those with even a passing interest in this new trend, you're not alone.

As I mentioned at the start of this book, ever since the WHI – the Women's Health Initiative study – announced the results of its mega trial some 6 years ago, more and more women have been turning away from traditional hormone replacement therapy. As you read earlier, it was during these studies that we first learned of many of the dangers and health concerns linked to HRT – as well as discovering that some of the benefits, such as protection from heart disease, didn't really prove true. And while for some women, low dose hormone therapy for a short period of time can still prove helpful in getting over that "hot flash" bump in the road, for the vast majority of us, the dangers of HRT far outweigh the benefits, particularly for long term use.

As a result, many women have taken a much greater interest in the use of natural or "bioidentical" hormones. But it's not just women themselves who are interested – some doctors are also taking notice of these treatments as well.

Indeed, out of from the ashes of the WHI trial an interesting question emerged. Namely, are all hormone treatments alike?

In fact, after the results of the WHI study was revealed, one question that frequently arose was whether or not the results would have been any different had other types of hormone based treatments been used. Some say yes.

Among the alternative treatments generating the greatest interest: Bioidentical or "natural" hormones – weaker forms of estrogen and progesterone garnered primarily from plant sources. Much like the effects of isoflavones found in the foods you read about earlier, many believe that when processed into a hormone treatment, plant estrogens harbor the same "curative" powers as synthetic hormones, without any of the negatives – such as an increased risk of certain cancers, stroke, or some forms of heart disease.

Adding more fuel to the speculative fires, celebrities like Suzanne Somers and more recently, Oprah Winfrey, as well as many naturopathic doctors made a great case for the benefits of natural hormones – believing that the results of the WHI would indeed have been different, had these nature-based hormonal compounds been used instead.

And, for many women these natural compounds do prove to work well, ameliorating not only hot flashes, but also a variety of other symptoms.

But that said, in the midst of all the excitement, a few basic but important facts seemed to be lost along the way. Among the most important: Whether or not these natural compounds are really any safer in the long run, then the traditional hormones we now fear.

The answer just might surprise you!

## FINDING THE TRUTH ABOUT NATURAL HORMONES

Among the first and most important facts to recognize is that while these "bioidentical" hormones are garnered from plant sources, putting them in the "natural" category can be a bit misleading. Indeed, unlike "natural" juice squeezed from an orange, no one is squeezing estrogen from a plant. Indeed, the process used to create bioidentical or natural hormone treatments is very similar to that used to create traditional "synthetic" hormone therapies. Both must undergo certain chemical processes in a laboratory in order to convert them into treatments.

Interestingly, some of the traditional "synthetic" hormones- treatments like Premarin and Provera - are also gleaned from "natural" substances and converted in a lab into hormone treatments. So, in this respect, words like "natural" don't hold a whole lot of meaning.

For many experts, however, the real difference between the new bioidentical hormones and the old-school traditional "synthetic" variety comes down to a matter of molecular structure.

Without getting too technical here, this means that on a molecular level, synthetic forms of estrogen and progesterone (like Provera or Premarin) are similar to, but not identical to the estrogen and progesterone produced in your body. Think of it as a copy of a designer dress – it can be very much *like* the original, but *not the original.*

By comparison, "natural" or "bioidentical" plant derived estrogens and progesterone *are identical – on a molecular level* – to what your body produces. Think designer original down to the last thread!

Now, will your body know the difference between the designer original – and the copy? Well, as in fashion, so goes it with hormones. For some women, it may make no difference at all. But for others, it could make a huge difference in how well the treatments are tolerated and whether or not symptoms are relieved.

The bigger question however is will that *small difference* in molecular structure make any *big difference* when it comes to health risks? And here is where the debate really heats up – the answer, very dependent upon whom you ask.

According to Wulf Utian, MD, executive director of the North American Menopause Society (NAMS), there is no question that bioidentical hormones hold little or no promise – and no advantages at all from the standpoint of health risks.

"The word Bioidentical is a marketing misnomer – and the claims for safety and efficacy are entirely without merit – they are the same as [synthetic] hormones and if given in bio-equivalent doses the risks would be exactly the same," he says.

Further he points out that any dosage which is strong enough to elicit a response and tame a symptom – like a hot flash – is strong enough to, at least potentially, cause harm.

But New York physician and long time proponent of natural hormones Erika Schwartz, MD sees it differently.

"When you change the molecular structure of a hormone – as is the case with synthetic hormones - then the body does not know what to do with it; conversely, when you give a supplement identical to what the body produces, then it knows exactly how to use it for the best possible advantage," says Schwartz.

In essence, Dr. Schwartz believes that because the body knows how to handle the bioidentical substances, many of the health risks associated with synthetic hormones, such as an increased risk of breast or ovarian cancer, or a stroke, won't be a threat when natural treatments are used.

The problem with that logic, however, is that we just don't know if the health risks associated with synthetic hormones are linked to the synthetic molecular structure – or if the introduction of hormones, in any form, at a time when our levels are naturally meant to decline may be what the health risks are really all about.

And the importance of this question is that right now, there is no answer. In truth, we don't really know if adding natural hormones into the menopausal mix will yield any fewer health risks than those linked to synthetic hormones, *because natural hormones have not been tested.*

That sentence is so important I'm going to say it again: *Natural hormones have not been tested* – at least not on the grand scale that traditional HRT has been studied. This becomes even more significant when you realize that once upon a time, we all believed that traditional HRT was our saving grace – a menopause panacea with no significant health risks and only health benefits.

In fact, forty or fifty years ago there were as many zealots proclaiming the benefits of HRT as there are bands of celebrity followers proclaiming the benefits of natural hormones today.

It wasn't, in fact, until we conducted the extensive WHI clinical trials that we found out just how wrong it was to assume traditional HRT was the answer, *before we had the proof.* It much the same way many believe it also seems wrong now to assume that natural hormones are the answer, when in fact, *we don't have the proof.*

Indeed, perhaps the most important lesson we learned from the WHI trials is that when it comes to women's health, let's not assume anything before we have the medical evidence to back up our beliefs.

And so now, it seems, we are at that very crossroads when it comes to natural or bio-identical hormones. We assume the naturals are better for us, and we assume that bio-identical hormones are safe.

But without the gold standard large-scale randomized placebo controlled clinical testing, how do we know for sure?

Well, we don't know. And until we do, using these preparations is a lot like riding a covered wagon through the old west – you don't really know what you're going to find what you get to your destination.

Will the fact that these hormones mimic exactly what the body produces be the saving grace that keeps us healthy?

Will it actually stop our hot flashes, without causing us harm? Or, like traditional HRT will they turn out to cause more problems than they solve?

Could it be, in fact, that pumping up our body with hormones at a time when nature decides they should decline will always yield bad results – even if those hormones come from Mother Nature herself?

These are the questions that have stumped both experts and celebrities alike.

"We are, in many ways, in a no-data zone - bio identical hormones have not been specifically studied in a randomized trial on any wide spread level, and if you are to use that as a criteria, then it's true that we don't know if they are any better- or any worse – than synthetic hormones," says Marcie Richardson, MD, Clinical instructor, Obstetrics and Gynecology at Harvard Medical School, and the director of the Menopause Consultation Service at Harvard Vanguard Medical Associates.

The one thing that is important to recognize however, is that science has already shown us that the more estrogen stimulation a woman has over her lifetime, the more likely she is to develop certain cancers, particularly breast cancer.

Indeed, women who have an early start to their menstrual cycle or continue to menstruate into their 50's are at greater risk for some female cancers. So too are women who have never had children. This is because being pregnant actually prevents ovulation – and estrogen-related ovarian stimulation – for at least 9 months.

We also know that women who are overweight are at greater risk for certain female cancers – and one reason may be because fat cells produce a form of "endogenous" estrogen. The more fat cells you have, the more estrogen stimulation you maintain, even after menopause occurs.

Does all this mean that after a certain number of years, estrogen stimulation of any kind – including that from bioidentical hormones or even our own hormones – is dangerous to our health?

Again, without adequate placebo-controlled randomized testing, the truth is, *we just don't know.*

## COMPOUNDING THE PROBLEM

Complicating matters just a bit more is the issue of how bio identical hormones are created and dispensed. While there are some FDA approved, pharmaceutical grade bio identical hormones (such as Prometrium, a natural progesterone, as well as bioidentical estrogens such as Estrace, Vivelle-Dot, Climara, Estring, and Vagifem), most of the "natural" preparations being touted by celebrities are prepared in very small batches by drugstores known as *compounding pharmacies.*

"This is a pharmacy that uses raw ingredients – like progesterone powder obtained from a distributor – to make a specific bio identical prescription written by a doctor," says NYU Professor of Obstetrics and Gynecology, Steve Goldstein, MD.

The problem is, however, that most doctors are not as familiar with writing formulations for these treatments as they might be in prescribing a pill that is already made. This means that in many instances, the doctors themselves must rely on the compounding pharmacies to suggest the dosages and combinations of various hormone components that ultimately end up in your prescription bottle. And that too has some experts very worried.

"They are making concoctions by adding in estriol, DHEA and other hormones, often at their own discretion – and even if they are filling what is being written in their opinion, who is checking batch to batch - no one, and it's just like practicing medicine without a license," says Utian.

While Richardson says compounding isn't always a bad thing – suggesting that when done responsibly it allows women the opportunity of individualized dosing - she does caution that quality control can become an issue.

Indeed, a recent study conducted by the FDA revealed up to 40% of drugs made in compounding pharmacies don't contain what they say they do. Utian says that in up to 10% of those drugs, the compounds contain 50% more of the active ingredient than what was on the prescription pad.

Are there good, reliable compounding pharmacies? Most definitely.  But again, even if the pharmacy represents utmost quality, the prescription you are getting is based more on their personal experience - and less on proven, scientifically scrutinized protocol. So again, without testing and now, without guaranteed quality control, trusting your symptoms to "natural" hormones might not be as comforting a choice as it should be.

## A Word About Hormone Testing

When it comes to using natural hormones you may also find that many compounding pharmacies as well as some naturopathic physicians advocate a number of blood and saliva tests as part of the prescribing profile. The tests measure amounts of specific hormones circulating through your blood and are used in an attempt to determine a more accurate natural hormone prescription – particularly in regard to dosing.

As good as this sounds, it's important to know that the use of these tests is even more controversial than the use of the hormone therapy itself – with some experts claiming they are virtually useless.

"A woman's hormones can change dramatically from hour to hour, as well as through her cycle and from cycle to cycle – there is absolutely nothing useful you can tell about a woman's menopause status from a hormone test – it's a waste of time and money and it's nonsense," says Utian.

That said, registered pharmacist Suzy Cohen, R.Ph, author of *The 24 Hour Pharmacist,* believes the tests are good under certain circumstances.

"The saliva tests are good for people who apply hormones right into their skin [such as via hormone creams]," she says, adding that it's essential to take the saliva test about midway between application doses for the most accurate results.

If you apply your hormone cream once a night – at say 10pm, Cohen says do your saliva test about 12 hours later, around 10am. If your reading is very high, she says you're using too much of the hormone cream. Or, you might be testing at the wrong time – so vary your testing time by several hours before changing your dosage.

Cohen also recommends a test known as the "Capillary Blood Spot", as way a helping to understand how well your natural hormone treatments are working.

This involves a painless finger prick that Cohen says shows "a very accurate picture of what is happening in your cells." And that may give you a more accurate picture of how well your hormone treatments are working.

If you're taking an oral form of hormones the most accurate reflection may be seen in a 24-hour urine test. Here you collect your urine for 24 hours and bring the sample to the lab or doctor, where it can be analyzed for hormone excretions. But don't try this on your own. You'll need a specially prepared container from the laboratory to keep the urine preserved until the sample can get to the laboratory.

You can find more information on the pros and cons of hormone testing and the use of natural hormones in my book *Your Perfectly Pampered Menopause,* or visit www.YourMenopause.com.

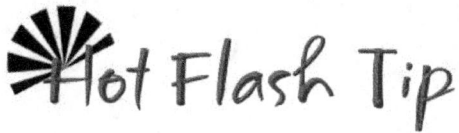

### Sunscreen and Hot Flashes

Do you notice that every time you put on sun screen
you get a hot flash? If so, you're not alone.
Many women find that as mid life approaches
chemicals found in most sunscreens suddenly
begin to irritate their skin , making their face feel
warm, and in some instances, exacerbate or even
ignite a hot flash.

While using a sun screen remains important, if you
think yours might be causing problems,
do try a different brand.
Sometimes even slight variations in formulations
can make a huge difference.

Also be aware that many foundations also contain
sunscreen – and they too can cause a facial flush.  If
you find that your face repeatedly gets warm within
5 to 20 minutes after applying your foundation, check
to see if it contains sunscreen. If you determine that
this is one of your hot flash triggers, look into natural,
mineral based make up which offers sunscreen
protection without harsh chemicals.  Brands least
likely to seep into fine lines and wrinkles include
Jane Iredale, Isadora and Glo Minerals.

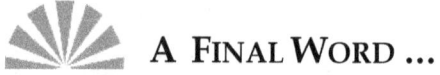

## A Final Word ...

# It's Your Menopause – Have It Your Way!

I am hopeful that what you have learned in this book will help make your life easier – and your menopause easier to endure. And I am very certain that as you go forward with the **Hot Flash Solutions Lifestyle Diary** you will begin to uncover even more ways to not only have fewer hot flashes and night sweats, but to feel better overall.

If you haven't already visited my blog, RedDressDiary.com or the companion website found at YourMeonpause.com, then I hope you'll stop by soon. Not only will you find the latest information on coping with all sorts of menopause symptoms, you'll also find some great advice on everything midlife, from skin care to hair care, make-up, fashion and style advice, nutrition, diet, exercise – it's all there!

But if you do stop by, you'll also find something else - something equally as important as a *Hot Flash Solution*. And that is, a healthy dose of midlife philosophy – one that embraces the "change" as a positive and not a negative life experience. Because the truth is, no matter what you've heard about this time of life, I can promise you that this is *not your mother's menopause* – not from a solutions standpoint and definitely not from a cultural point of view.

Want to know just how our views have changed in the last 30 years?

Remember that wonderful 1970's show, "All InThe Family" …with Archie Bunker and his doting, housecoat clad, sensible shoe-wearing wife Edith, brilliantly played by actress Jean Stapleton.

Keep her in mind as you fast-forward to the 1990's and the sassy, steamy, show *Sex and the City* and the salty, sexy Samantha – brilliantly portrayed by Kim Cattrall.

What do these two shows – and these two women - have in common? I hope you're sitting down: The sexy siren Samantha and the doting housewife Edith … *were roughly the same age!* And both, at some point in their respective shows – went through menopause!

That's just one example of *how much* things have changed! Indeed, today women are living longer – and healthier – than ever before, and the *temporary* interruption we call menopause, well, it's really just a blip on the radar screen of your life. When you exit on the other side of that hot flash I can promise there's is a whole new world waiting to be discovered…by you!

Of course if you hang on to the idea that all your hopes and dreams are floating away on a sea of hot flashes and night sweats, well, they just might. But if you embrace this time in your life with the same fervor you did other major life changes – like marriage or pregnancy, your college graduation or your career successes – then I promise your life will take on a new dimension and a new meaning, and possibly the best you've ever known.

So don't buy into those old stereotypes of what menopause means – or for that matter, what being 50, 60, 70 or more really means. If you have dreams yet to fulfill, things you want to accomplish in life – this is the time to go for it! Many of the fears and worries you had in your youth will melt away during this time of life – giving you the chance to once again find yourself and your dreams.

As I leave you for the moment, I leave you with my favorite RedDressDiary quote:

### "BEAUTY IS AGELESS, SUCCESS IS AGELESS, FALLING IN LOVE IN AGELESS."

Be good to yourself …and to each other! And please drop me a line & let me know just how menopause is changing your life for the better!

Warmest regards;

*Colette Bouchez*

# YOUR MENOPAUSE REFERENCE LIBRARY

## Extra Resources to Learn Even More!

### Newsletters, Magazines, and Web Sites

- **RedDressDiary**
- www.RedDressDiary.com

- **YourMenopause.com**
  www.YourMenopause.com

- **Healthy Women Today**
  http://www.womenshealth.gov/newsletter/
- 
  **Menopause Flashes**
  http://www.menopause.org/newsletter.htm

### Government Agencies

- **Womenshealth.gov, OWH, HHS \***
  www.womenshealth.gov/menopause
- 
- **Office on Women's Health, HHS**
  http://www.womenshealth.gov/owh
- 
- **Administration on Aging, HHS**
  http://www.aoa.dhhs.gov

•**National Center for Complementary and Alternative Medicine, NIH, HHS \***
http://nccam.nih.gov
•

•**Office of Research on Women's Health, NIH, HHS**
http://orwh.od.nih.gov/index.html
•

•**Office of Women's Health, CDC, HHS**
http://www.cdc.gov/women/
•

•**Office of Women's Health, FDA, HHS**
http://www.fda.gov/womens/default.htm
•

•**Osteoporosis and Related Bone Diseases National Resource Center, NIH, HHS \***
http://www.osteo.org

**Private Organizations**

•**American College of Obstetricians and Gynecologists (ACOG) (Offers Publications in Spanish)**
http://www.acog.org
•

•**American Menopause Foundation, Inc. (Offers**
http://www.americanmenopause.org
•

•**Black Women's Health Imperative**
http://www.blackwomenshealth.org
•

•**Boston Women's Health Book Collective (Offers publications in Spanish)**
http://www.ourbodiesourselves.org

•**Hormone Foundation** *
http://www.hormone.org
•

•**The Jean Mayer USDA Human Nutrition Research Center on Aging**
http://hnrc.tufts.edu
•

•**National Osteoporosis Foundation (NOF)**
http://www.nof.org
•

•**National Women's Health Network**
http://www.nwhn.org
•

•**North American Menopause Society (NAMS) (Offers publications in Spanish)**
http://www.menopause.org

BOOKS:

YOUR PERFECTLY PAMPERED MENOPAUSE BY COLETTE BOUCHEZ    (BROADWAY BOOKS, NY )

•COULD IT BE PERIMENOPAUSE BY STEVEN GOLDSTEIN, MD

•THE WISDOM OF MENOPAUSE BY CHRISTIANE NORTHRUP, MD

•THE 24-HOUR PHARMACIST BY SUZY COHEN, R.PH

# About Colette Bouchez

## *Author of "The Hot Flash Solution"*

Colette Bouchez is a nationally recognized healthy *lifestyle expert,* an award winning medical journalist for over two decades and the author of 8 books on women's wellness.

Formerly the content producer for women's health at WebMD and the former senior medical reporter for the New York Daily News her experience in reporting and writing about women's health issues spans more than two decades.

Ms. Bouchez's work has been honored by many leading medical organizations including:

- The American Cancer Society
- The American Academy of Dermatology
- The American College of Colon Surgeons
- The Coalition of Breast Cancer Organizations
- The Multiple Sclerosis Society

In 1996 she was the writer in the award winning WNBC TV- Daily News team that produced a 7-day report on breast cancer, taking the Emmy for best news documentary.

In addition to professional journalism memberships, in 2001 Colette Bouchez became one of only a handful of journalists admitted to the prestigious AMWA -American Medical Women's Association - the division of the American Medical Association that honors female physicians and researchers.

Colette Bouchez is the creator and founder of YourMenopause.com, and the RedDressDiary.com – an online column and website dedicated to helping women over 40 lead a happier, healthier, more beautiful life! It's where you'll find the very best, the very latest health, beauty and lifestyle information available for your age group.

Write Colette at: RedDressDiary@aol.com

**Other books by Colette Bouchez include:**

**Your Perfectly Pampered Menopause**
**Health, Beauty, Life & Style**
**For The Best Years of Your Life**
(Broadway Books-Random House)

**Your Perfectly Pampered Pregnancy**
*Beauty, Health, and Style for the*
*Modern Mother-To-Be*
(Broadway Books – Random House)

**The V Zone**
*A Woman's Guide To Intimate Health*
*(Fireside – Simon & Schuster)*

**Getting Pregnant:**
*What You Need To Know Now*
*(Fireside- Simon & Schuster)*

If you loved The Hot Flash Solution,

you'll  positively, absolutely love, love, love

Your Perfectly Pampered Menopause:

Health, Beauty, Life & Style Advice

For the Best Years of Your Life!

By Colette Bouchez

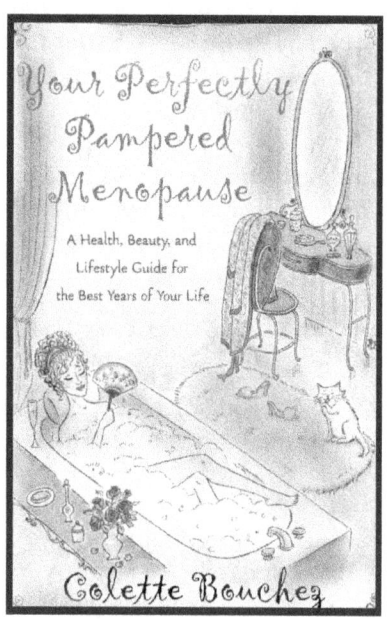

www.YourMenopause.com

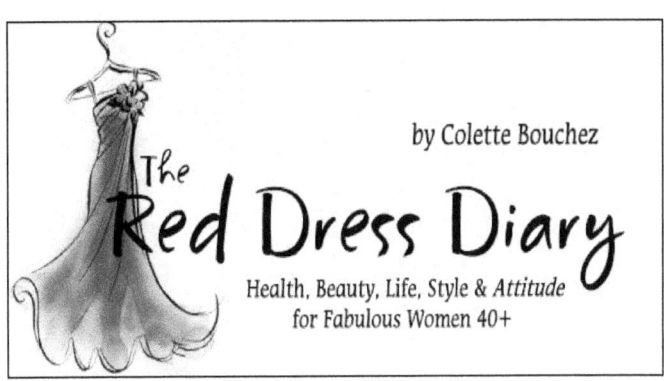
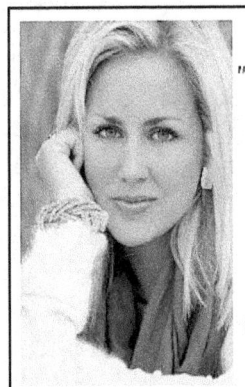